MUCUNA Vademecum
(User guide for Parkinson's disease)

Dr Rafael Gonzalez Maldonado,
neurologist

2

Mucuna Vademecum

(User guide for Parkinson's disease)

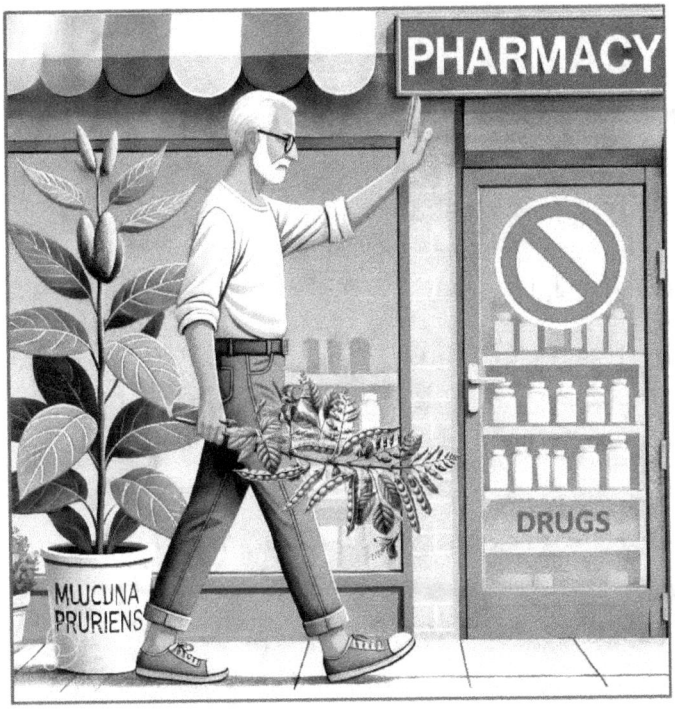

Dr Rafael Gonzalez Maldonado,
neurologist

Title : Mucuna Vademecum

Subtitle: Parkinson's user guide

Author : Rafael Gonzalez Maldonado

Collaboration (chap. 11): Marianne van der Meer, Jérôme Simonin.

Publisher: KDP Amazon, North Charleston

1st EDITION, September 2024

2nd EDITION, November 2024

This English edition has been revised by Jérôme Simonin MA (translator spec. in Medical English)

KDP ISBN: 9798340774286

©Copyright 2024 : Rafael Gonzalez Maldonado

All rights reserved, rafael@gonzalezmaldonado.com

WARNING: The concepts and data in this book are not medical recommendations, but rather suggestions that are questionable and subject to error. Patients and their caregivers should always follow the advice of their physician.

To Rafael, Jaime, Alvaro, Julio, Claudia and Carlos

I have prolonged the echo of blood to which I respond
(MIGUEL HERNÁNDEZ, *Wind of the people*, 1937)

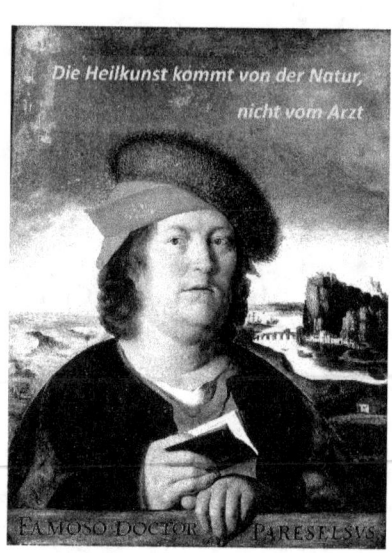

"The art of healing comes from nature, not from the physician. Therefore, the physician must start from nature, with an open mind." *

(PARACELSUS 1493-1541)

---

*"Die Heilkunst kommt von der Natur, nicht vom Arzt. Deshalb muss der Arzt von der Natur ausgehen, mit einem offenen Geist." (PARACELSUS)

Index

Introduction

1. Mucuna is more than just levodopa
2. The "mucuna of the poor"
3. The "Internet mucuna"
4. Pure powder of the plant or its seeds
5. Low-concentrated extracts
6. Medium-concentrated extracts
7. Ultra-concentrated extracts
8. Elixirs of mucuna
9. How to start with mucuna!
10. How to add mucuna to the treatment!
11. Patients lose their patience (Patient forum)
12. Mucuna preparation tables

Bibliography

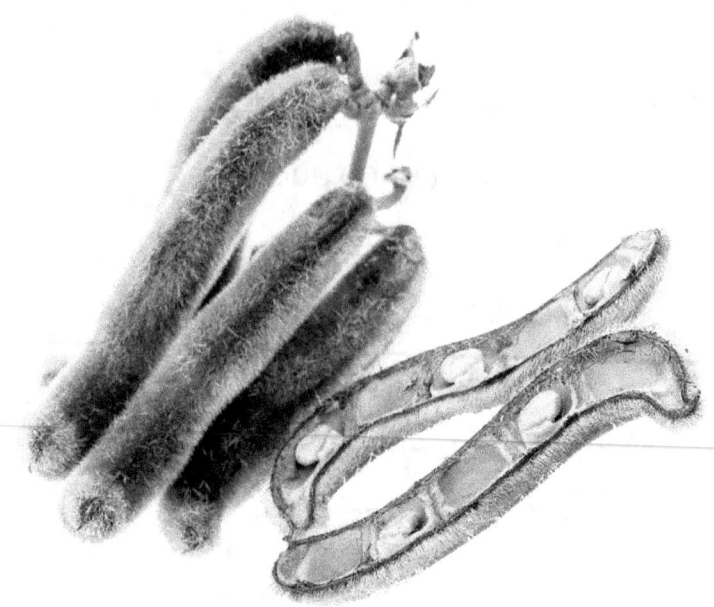

Mucuna pruriens

Introduction

Mucuna pruriens is a tropical bean with a high levodopa content, which is why it is used as a complementary (not alternative) treatment for Parkinson's disease. Unfortunately, it is not very well known by the patients who take it or even the doctors who prescribe or prohibit it.

It can be confusing because there are so many products out there containing mucuna, and not all of them have the right instructions. Sometimes, they do not even contain what they promise!

Formulations can be rather complex, and they often depend on the part of the plant used, the preparation method, the concentration and the presentation (like powder, capsules, elixirs, and so on). It can be confusing to accurately estimate the amount of natural levodopa being ingested. It is also difficult to predict how well it will work in practice. The good news is that symptoms can be improved, but it is important to remember that this is only a quarter of the improvement seen with conventional levodopa preparations, which include carbidopa or benserazide to enhance the effect.

It is also important to remember that other factors like the way your body processes levodopa, the bacteria in your gut, and what you eat can all affect how you respond to treatment.

If a patient who was only taking mucuna adds a drug such as Sinemet or Madopar, the effect of levodopa on their body could be multiplied by four, which could lead to some unwanted side effects.

In this book, we're delighted to analyse the most popular brands, unraveling their often confusing formulations and precisely calculating the amount of levodopa they contain.

We have also sections on pure seed powder, and on the advantages of encapsulating it for those who find its taste unpleasant.

In other chapters, we will have a look at mucuna extracts in powder or capsule form, with different degrees of concentration: low potency (10-20%), medium potency (40-60%) and ultra-concentrated (more than 90% levodopa).

We will also discuss other ways to take levodopa, such as liquid elixirs and other products that are a little different, mentioning those with piperine (which comes from black pepper) or gummy presentations that you can take under your tongue. These help levodopa get into your blood faster because they avoid going through your intestines. We will also talk about some interesting combinations of simple stem extracts with seed concentrates!

And finally, we have included a practical guide with examples on how to use mucuna and recommendations on the most appropriate presentations and concentrations for you, depending on where you are in your Parkinson's journey.

For more, see my other books on mucuna and Parkinson's: *Mucuna against Parkinson's*, *Natural remedies for Parkinson's disease*, and *Ecological treatment of Parkinson's disease*.

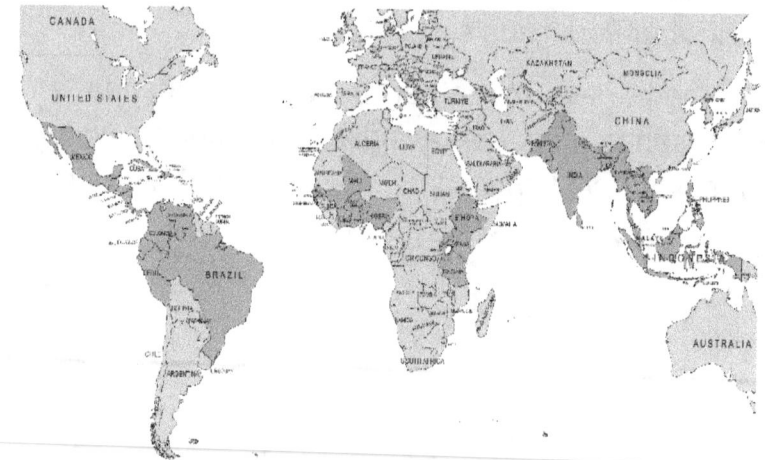

FIGURE 1: Mucuna pruriens is a bean that grows in tropical regions and contains a lot of natural levodopa.

Its seeds, in powder or extract form, are the most effective natural product for treating Parkinson's disease.

1. Mucuna is more than just levodopa

Mucuna pruriens is the scientific name of a tropical bean, which is also known as velvet bean, *kapicatchu* or *pica-pica*. This amazing plant has been used in Ayurvedic medicine for more than 3,000 years to help with Parkinson's disease (kampavata) and other ailments.

The seeds are packed with levodopa, which is a precursor to dopamine. This is a neurotransmitter that is often low in people with Parkinson's disease. It is so fantastic to see more and more interest in mucuna! Its natural levodopa content is exciting because it seems to offer some amazing therapeutic advantages over synthetic forms.

THE PLANT

Mucuna is a lovely legume, a type of bean that grows in tropical regions of Africa, Asia and the Caribbean. Its seeds are packed with levodopa, with an enormous 3% to 7% content! That is the highest natural levodopa content found in a plant.

In traditional Ayurvedic medicine, it is highly valued not only for its levodopa content, but also as an aphrodisiac and for other beneficial properties (PATHAK 2017).

Exciting new studies show that Mucuna pruriens is packed with more than just levodopa – it also possesses rather impressive compounds like serotonin, nicotine and antioxidants, which suggest it could be a real healing powerhouse! (BOONMONGKOL 2019).

UNKNOWN COMPONENTS IN MUCUNA

The therapeutic potential of *Mucuna pruriens* extends beyond its levodopa content. Several studies demonstrate a complex phytochemical profile that remains to be understood. More than 50 bioactive compounds have been identified in the seeds, and some could promote the absorption and metabolism of levodopa, improve motor symptoms and even act as neuroprotectants. They contain alkaloids, glycoproteins and phytochemicals (prurienin, mucunin), which are presumed to act synergistically with levodopa to alleviate parkinsonian symptoms and may explain why mucuna is often more effective and better tolerated than synthetic levodopa alone.

IMPROVEMENTS IN MICE

Studies in animal models of Parkinson's disease have shown promising results. In mice, mucuna outperformed synthetic levodopa in improving motor function, doubling or tripling the beneficial effects. Neuroprotective effects have also been observed in rodents, such as preservation of dopaminergic neurons and reduction of oxidative stress.

HUMAN IMPROVEMENTS

Researchers have compared mucuna to Sinemet and Madopar and have shown that patients taking mucuna experience faster symptom relief, higher blood levels of levodopa, and longer duration of effects. They also experience fewer side effects, such as dyskinesia, a common complication of long-term synthetic levodopa treatment.

As an example, four human clinical trials:

Study 1: A traditional, very effective preparation

It was pioneered in 1995 by Manyan and the Parkinson Study Group. 60 patients diagnosed with Parkinson's disease were recruited, 26 of them were taking synthetic levodopa/ carbidopa medications, while the remaining 34 were levodopa naïve. For 12 weeks, patients were given a traditional Ayurvedic medicine product (HP-200) in powder form, developed from traditional Ayurvedic medicine (similar to Zandopa seed powder), mixed with water and consumed orally. Symptoms were assessed with the Unified Parkinson's Disease Rating Scale (UPDRS).

UPDRS scores and Hoehn and Yahr stage were very significantly reduced (<0.0001, t-test), indicating an improvement in motor symptoms and quality of life of patients. The optimal mean daily dose to control symptoms was 6 ± 3 sachets: that is, 3 to 9 sachets (each containing 7.5 grams of seed powder) = between 22 and 67 grams/day.* Side effects were mild and mainly gastrointestinal, such as stomach upset or nausea. These results suggest that natural compounds, such as mucuna, may offer an alternative or complement to conventional treatments.

Study 2: Rapid and lasting improvement

A 2004 study by Katzenschlager compared Mucuna pruriens with conventional levodopa/carbidopa (LD/CD) treatment in patients with advanced Parkinson's disease. Eight participants received both options in a crossover design. The results:

- Rapid action: mucuna showed a faster onset than LD/CD, with noticeable effects in 34 minutes compared to 68 minutes for conventional levodopa.

- Longer duration: MP effects lasted 22% longer, prolonging the time in the " on " state, when symptoms improve.

- Reduced dyskinesias: No significant increase in involuntary movements was observed, indicating a favourable safety profile.

---

*Estimating a levodopa content of 3.3%, that means between 740 and 2,227 mg of levodopa.

This study showed that mucuna could be more effective than standard levodopa, providing faster and longer lasting relief without increasing side effects.

Study 3: Comparison of high and low doses

In 2017, Cilia and team evaluated 18 patients with advanced PD (CILIA 2017), administering high and low doses of mucuna together with LD/CD. High dose Mucuna pruriens showed significant improvement in motor symptoms at 90 and 180 minutes, with a longer duration of the "on" state (45 additional minutes) compared to LD/CD. There were fewer dyskinesias compared to conventional treatment. These results suggest that Mucuna, at adequate doses, is not only comparable to synthetic levodopa, but might offer better tolerance to side effects and greater long-term safety.

Study 4: High doses in advanced patients.

A 16-week trial published in 2018 (CILIA 2018) evaluated the tolerability and efficacy of mucuna when used daily in patients with advanced Parkinson's disease. Fourteen patients alternated between MP and LD/CD to measure their clinical response.

Half of the patients were unable to continue MP due to gastrointestinal side effects or motor impairment but were able to continue with a water-diluted form. In those who tolerated it, the clinical effects were comparable to those of LD/CD.

Conclusion: human clinical studies have shown that mucuna is an effective and safe alternative to synthetic levodopa in the treatment of advanced Parkinson's disease. Its rapid onset and long-lasting effect, together with a lower risk of dyskinesias, make it particularly attractive.

OTHER ADVANTAGES OF MUCUNA

Mucuna offers other important advantages, such as not increasing the risk of dyskinesia with prolonged use, a common limitation of synthetic levodopa. In animal models, prolonged use of mucuna does not produce dyskinesias, an important limitation of synthetic levodopa. It also has neuroprotective properties, probably due to its high antioxidant content, which may slow the progression of Parkinson's. In addition, it does not seem to require a constant increase in dosage, making it a more sustainable option in the long term.

QUADRUPLE THE DOSE

Mucuna has clear advantages, but since it does not contain carbidopa, in order to achieve symptomatic improvement to the same level as synthetic levodopa preparations containing carbidopa (or benserazide), the amount of natural levodopa must be four times that of synthetic levodopa (between 2.5 and 4.5 times, to be more precise).

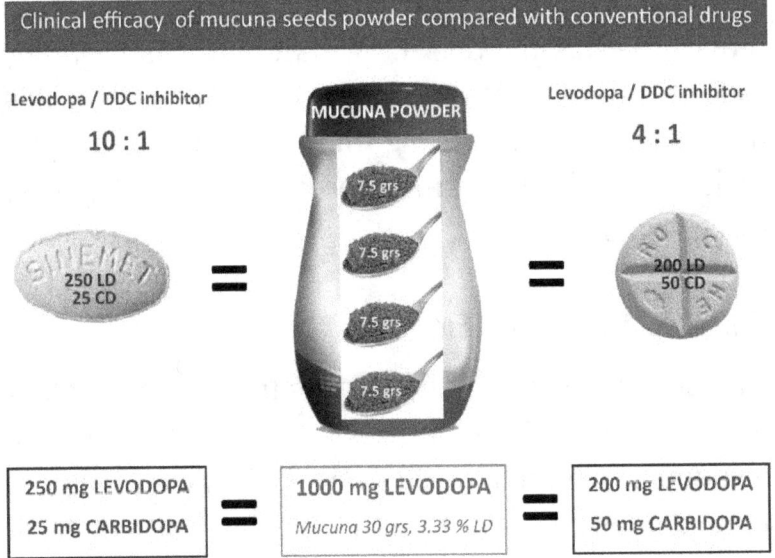

Thus, to achieve the same clinical efficacy as a Sinemet 25/250 tablet (25 mg of carbidopa and 250 mg of levodopa), 1000 mg of mucuna levodopa (30 grams of simple seed powder, without extracts) must be given.

This rate of improvement varies depending on the individual profile, the way a person metabolizes levodopa, their intestinal microbiota, diet, and the presence of other medications.

MUCUNA WITH CARBIDOPA

Carbidopa is not available separately in Europe, but some researchers combined mucuna with carbidopa, a dopa-decarboxylase inhibitor (DANIQUE 2019). This greatly improved its efficacy by preventing peripheral degradation of levodopa, allowing a larger amount to reach the brain. This combination would greatly reduce the necessary dose of mucuna, while maintaining or improving the therapeutic effects, making the treatment more practical and with fewer side effects.

THE VOLUME PROBLEM

One challenge in using mucuna is the volume of plant material needed to obtain a therapeutic dose of levodopa. To match the efficacy of a standard Sinemet tablet, patients need to consume large amounts of mucuna, and that is impractical. However, recent advances in extraction and concentration techniques have made it possible to create more manageable doses in capsules or tablets.

PATENTS ON MUCUNA EXTRACTS

Specific extraction techniques and formulations of *Mucuna pruriens* have been patented for the treatment of Parkinson's disease. Applicants include renowned neurologists such as WC Olanow and AJ Lees (VAN DER GIESSEN 2004). These patents highlight the unique properties of Mucuna, not only for its levodopa content but also for its potential to protect neurons and alleviate other neurodegenerative conditions.

Compared to conventional levodopa, they found that *Mucuna* provides a wider therapeutic window, allowing effective treatment at lower doses with fewer side effects. Symptom relief is faster and more sustained, without increasing the risk of dyskinesias.

DYSKINESIAS DUE TO LEVODOPA OR CARBIDOPA?

Mucuna has natural levodopa, but no carbidopa. And to be effective it needs it, but not in the 1:4 ratio of Sinemet Plus 25/100, a smaller ratio would be enough, such as 1:10 of Sinemet 25/250, or perhaps even smaller: 1:15, 1:20...

What if carbidopa is the culprit of dyskinesias? I mean, too much carbidopa. This is suspected in some articles (HINZ 2014a and 2014b).

Mucuna has levodopa and if it does not cause dyskinesia, it is because it does not have carbidopa. But because it does not have carbidopa, its dose must be quadrupled to achieve a similar effect to Sinemet.

CONTRAINDICATIONS AND WARNINGS

Although Mucuna offers important therapeutic benefits, it shares contraindications with synthetic levodopa. It should be used with caution in patients with cardiovascular disease, psychosis, or those taking specific medications, such as MAO inhibitors.

With MAO inhibitors (MAOI) they can increase blood pressure. In those treated with anticoagulants and aspirin, the risk of bleeding increases. Mucuna lowers blood sugar somewhat, which is considered in diabetics. If combined with antiparkinsonian drugs, mucuna can enhance the effect of levodopa and others (which is sometimes sought). It can increase the demand for vitamins B1 and B6, so a low-dose supplement is recommended.

Since mucuna products lack regulation and standardization, medical supervision is essential to avoid adverse effects or unwanted interactions.

PATIENTS DO NOT KNOW WHAT THEY ARE TAKING

A major challenge in the use of mucuna is the lack of knowledge among patients, who often self-medicate without understanding the proper dosage or possible interactions with other medications.

Variability in levodopa content and lack of standardization between products may result in overdose or underdose. It is essential that patients consult their physician regularly to ensure proper dosage and avoid adverse interactions with other medications.

SKEPTICAL DOCTORS

Many doctors are still skeptical. This is due, in part, to the lack of large-scale clinical trials and the lack of knowledge about the plant in Western medicine. Other doctors allow their patients to use mucuna as a supplement, but do not intervene in the dosage, which is admittedly complicated by the variety of presentations and unclear formulations. This book aims to facilitate its understanding.

CONCLUSIONS

Mucuna is a promising natural alternative to synthetic levodopa for the treatment of Parkinson's disease. Its combination of levodopa and bioactive compounds provides benefits such as faster symptom relief, longer duration of effects, and lower risk of dyskinesia. Its use should be supervised by physicians to ensure its safety and efficacy.

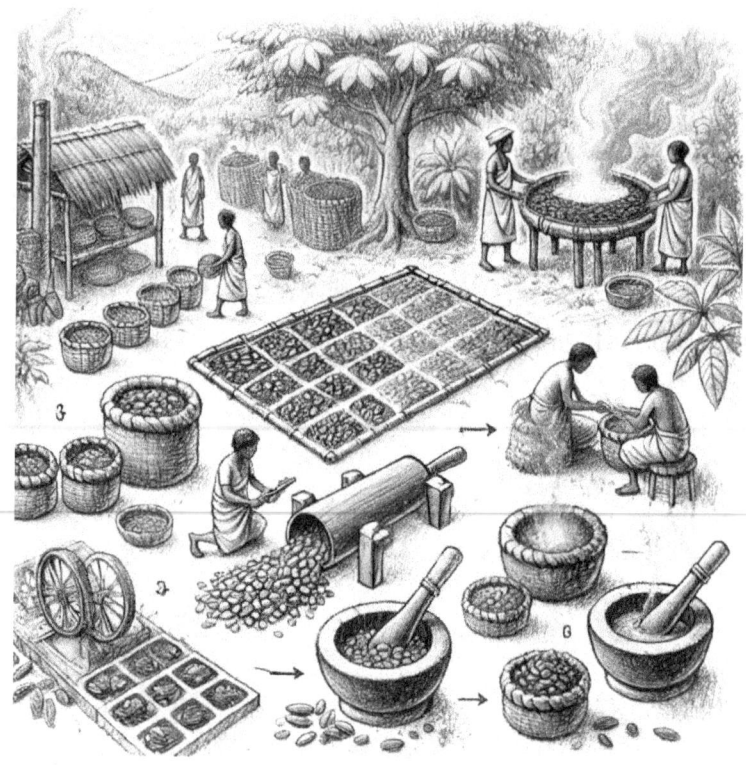

FIGURE 3: Natural process of making mucuna, as it has been done for millennia. In underdeveloped countries, mucuna is the alternative to treat people with Parkinson's disease,

2. The mucuna of the poor

In many ways, this "poor man's mucuna" is more complete than that consumed in developed countries although it also has its disadvantages.

CULTIVATION IN UNDERDEVELOPED COUNTRIES

Mucuna pruriens is widely cultivated in tropical and subtropical regions, with a particular focus on Africa, Asia and Latin America. Countries such as India, Nigeria, Ghana, Uganda, Tanzania, Guatemala and Brazil value this plant for both its agricultural and medicinal benefits.

In these areas, mucuna grows spontaneously and is considered an invasive species due to its rapid growth. This means that its development does not require special care, which makes it easy to cultivate.

In countries such as Brazil and Ghana, it is integrated into sustainable agriculture systems, improving crop yields and protecting soil from erosion. Recent research has shown that mucuna is resistant to many pests and diseases, making it a very attractive option for farmers in resource-limited regions.

MEDICINAL USE

The medicinal use of Mucuna pruriens has been documented in several cultures, highlighting the treatment of Parkinson's disease and other neurological processes. The levodopa from its seeds is converted into dopamine in the brain and motor symptoms are controlled in patients with Parkinson's.

PREPARATION TO ELIMINATE TOXINS

Mucuna contains natural toxins, such as serotonin and bufotenin, which must be removed before consumption. Traditional techniques include:

1. Washing and soaking: in many cultures, mucuna seeds are washed and soaked in water for several hours or days, thereby reducing soluble toxins.

2. Prolonged cooking: after soaking, the seeds are boiled for a long time, which is crucial to break down other toxins.

3. Fermentation and roasting: in some cases, the seeds are fermented or roasted. Roasting at 150°C for 15 minutes, followed by decortication, has been shown to be effective in reducing toxins and preserving levodopa (CASSANI et al).

HEALTH EFFECTS AND SAFETY OF USE

Mucuna is effective in treating Parkinson's disease due to its high content of natural levodopa, accompanied by other bioactive compounds that may enhance its efficacy and reduce the common side effects associated with synthetic levodopa. It has a favorable pharmacokinetic profile that could reduce the risk and severity of dyskinesias (CASSANI et al.).

The concentration of levodopa in mucuna seeds varies depending on the preparation method, being higher in dried and roasted seeds than in boiled ones.

MUCUNA FOR POOR PATIENTS

Limited access to conventional drugs for the treatment of Parkinson's disease is a major problem in many developing countries. As mucuna grows abundantly in these regions, it is a viable and affordable alternative for the treatment of this disease.

In sub-Saharan Africa, where 60% of the population lives on less than $2 a day, the daily cost of levodopa treatment is about $1 (half a salary).

In contrast, 1 kg of mucuna seeds costs 1 USD, which is enough for 50 days of treatment at an average daily dose (CASSANI et al.). Evidently, mucuna could be a sustainable solution for Parkinson's patients in low-income countries (CARONNI 2024).

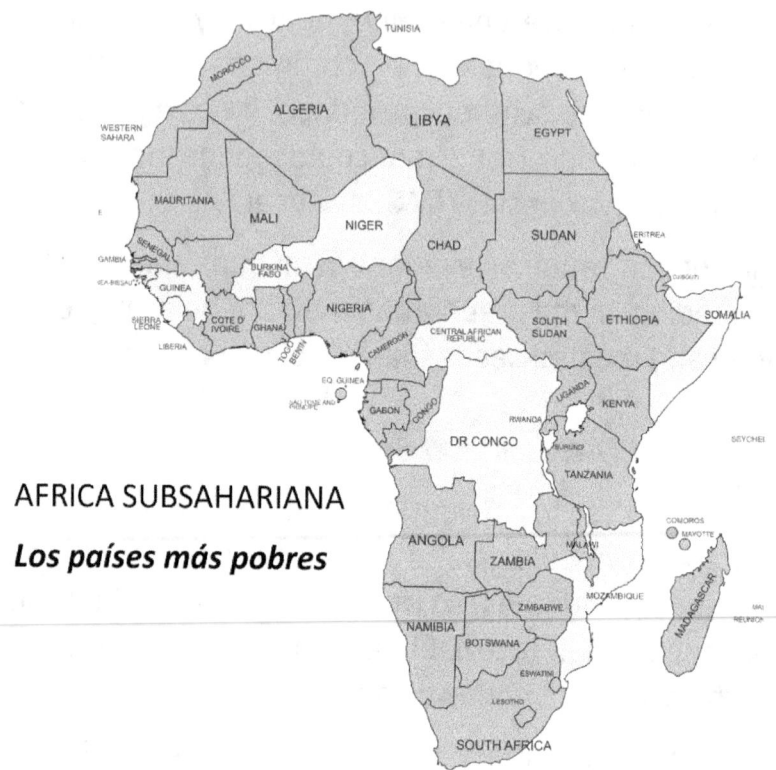

AFRICA SUBSAHARIANA

Los países más pobres

CONCLUSIONS

Mucuna pruriens is a plant of immense value in underdeveloped countries, not only for its agricultural applications, but also for its therapeutic potential in the treatment of Parkinson's disease.

Through traditional preparation techniques, mucuna becomes a safe, effective and accessible alternative to conventional medicines in resource-limited regions.

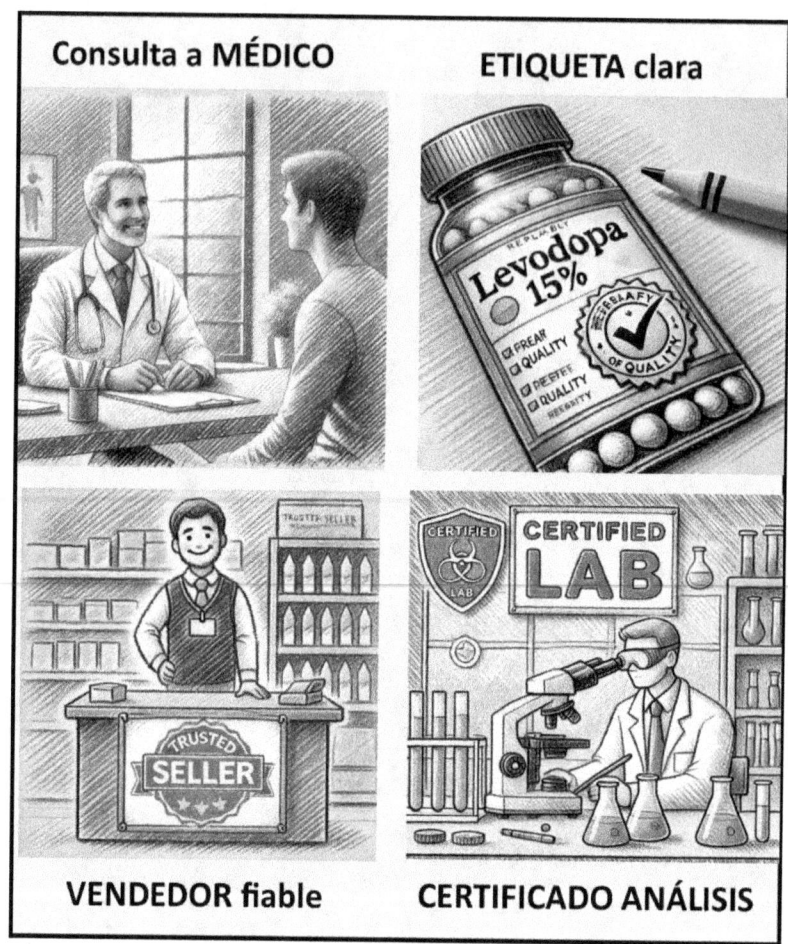

FIGURE 3: WHEN PURCHASING MUCUNA ONLINE
1. Consult a doctor
2. Reliable brands with clear labels
3. Reliable seller
4. Certificate of analysis

3. The Internet mucuna

In developed countries, laboratories that market mucuna adhere to rigorous safety and quality standards. However, some choose to employ more natural techniques to preserve the integrity and potency of this plant, known for its high content of levodopa, a precursor of dopamine vital for the treatment of Parkinson's disease.

SUSTAINABLE CROPS AND HARVESTING

Mucuna pruriens comes from crops in tropical and subtropical regions of Africa, Asia and Latin America, using organic farming methods.

These farming practices, which avoid the use of synthetic pesticides and fertilizers, ensure that plant material is free of chemical contaminants. In some areas, mucuna is grown in crop rotation and polyculture systems, which helps maintain soil health and reduces pesticide pressure.

TRADITIONAL AND MODERN PROCESSING

After harvest, mucuna seeds and plant material are sun-dried to preserve their active compounds.

The combination of traditional methods, such as sun drying and roasting, with modern extraction techniques, has proven to be highly effective in maintaining the quality of the final product , improving the bioavailability of certain bioactive compounds, increasing their therapeutic value.

In laboratories that produce mucuna without artificial extraction, traditional methods of decoction and infusion are used, together with modern techniques such as supercritical CO_2 extraction, which guarantee the obtaining of extracts with a high concentration of levodopa.

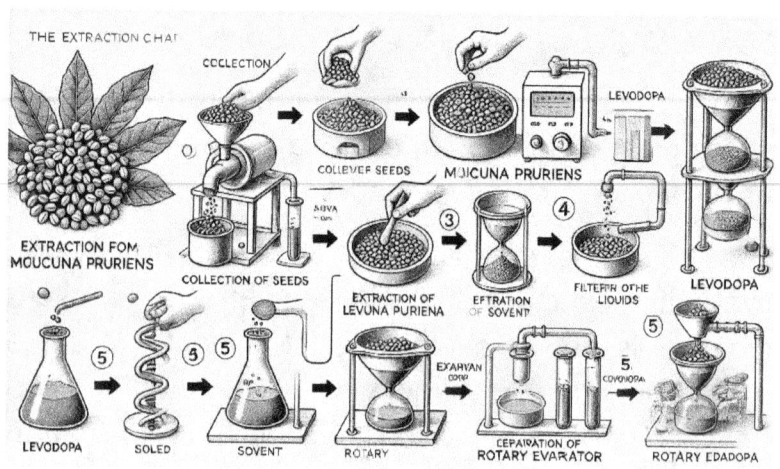

QUALITY CONTROL AND STANDARDIZATION

Quality control is a critical aspect in the production of Mucuna pruriens extracts. Laboratories employ advanced analytical techniques such as high-performance liquid chromatography (HPLC) and mass spectrometry to ensure that products are consistent and safe. These techniques allow key metabolites, such as levodopa, to be identified and quantified, ensuring that products meet international quality standards.

LEVODOPA VARIES ACCORDING TO PROCESSING

A recent study indicates that variations in processing methods can significantly affect the concentration of levodopa in mucuna seeds. In some regions, seeds collected from local markets showed variations in their levodopa content, underscoring the importance of standardization in the production of Mucuna products.

PACKAGING AND PRESERVATION

Mucuna products are packaged under controlled conditions to preserve their active compounds.

Using glass containers protects the product from light and air, factors that could degrade levodopa over time. In addition, some laboratories use advanced techniques such as freeze-drying, which helps maintain product stability for extended periods.

BIOTECHNOLOGY

Biotechnology plays a crucial role in optimizing the production of mucuna. Recent research has allowed to improve the cultivation conditions and the yield of bioactive compounds through genetic engineering.

In India, for example, mucuna varieties have been developed with higher concentrations of levodopa, which improves their therapeutic efficacy.

ETHICS AND FAIR TRADE

Many laboratories work in direct collaboration with local farmers, ensuring fair wages and sustainable farming practices. This collaboration not only supports the local economy, but also ensures the integrity of the supply chain, contributing to the production of high-quality, naturally processed mucuna products.

CONCENTRATED SEED EXTRACTS

Mucuna seeds are highly valued for their high concentration of levodopa. The seeds are carefully selected to ensure their ripeness and quality. In Bolivia and Ghana, the seeds undergo a roasting process that improves the bioavailability of certain compounds, thereby maximizing the therapeutic value of the final product.

EXTRACTION TECHNIQUES

The extraction process is critical to obtaining a high-quality product. Techniques such as supercritical CO_2 extraction and the use of ultrasound have proven to be highly efficient in obtaining pure and concentrated extracts. These techniques, combined with traditional methods, ensure that the extract contains the highest possible amount of levodopa and other beneficial compounds.

NORMALIZATION (STANDARDIZATION)

Standardization is crucial to ensure that each batch of mucuna extract has a consistent concentration of levodopa. Quality testing is performed to confirm the levodopa concentration and ensure that the extract meets international regulations. This is especially important in therapeutic applications such as the treatment of Parkinson's disease.

ENCAPSULATION AND FORMULATION

Concentrated mucuna extract is encapsulated or mixed with other ingredients for consumption, ensuring that each dose is safe and effective. Advanced packaging techniques are used to protect the product from external factors that could compromise its stability, such as light, air and moisture.

QUALITY CONTROL

Quality control is an essential aspect in the production of mucuna extracts. Rigorous tests are carried out to confirm the concentration of levodopa, the absence of contaminants and the stability of the product. These tests ensure that the extract complies with all the regulations necessary for its commercialization and is safe for consumption.

INTERNET SCAMS WITH MUCUNA

You will find *good* and *bad* mucunas on sale on the Internet. If the content and concentration of the formula are not clear, do not buy them. In addition, many lie by advertising a quantity of levodopa that they do not contain.

My colleague Tanya Denne (a researcher in Oregon) raised the alarm (SOUMYANATH 2018) after analyzing six mucuna products: three of the brands contained only 6, 34 or 40% of the levodopa declared on the packaging. Three others did contain the amount they claim and even more.

The researchers do not give the brand names, but I was able to identify them. I will not mention the defective ones, but those that live up to their promise: Dopabean (Solaray), Mucuna Dopa (Source Natural) and Zandopa (Zandu).

In autumn 2022, another analysis of 16 mucuna products (COHEN 2022) [6] showed huge variations in levodopa content: from 2 to 241 mg. If you buy mucuna, the leaflet is not enough, ask for a certificate of the content, which differentiates the amount of powder or seed extract, the percentage of levodopa and what each unit really contains (sometimes they give the value of levodopa per *dose,* which can be two capsules).

TIPS WHEN BUYING MUCUNA

If you are looking for mucuna as a complementary treatment, you should do your research and avoid the risks of low-quality or counterfeit supplements.

1. Consult your doctor. He or she can confirm whether the mucuna product is suitable for you, and will guide you on dosages, and monitor for drug interactions.

2. Reliable brands. Look for companies with a solid reputation and a track record of quality; that comply with "Good Manufacturing Practices" (GMP, and that have Quality Certifications from recognized organizations (FDA in the US, EMA in Europe, others).

3. Check the composition. Read the label carefully: it should clearly indicate the amount of levodopa per dose. Avoid those that give scant or dubious information about the content.

4. Independent analysis – Check whether third-party laboratories have confirmed the levodopa content, and that it is free of harmful contaminants such as heavy metals.

5. Learn from others' experiences. Read reviews and comments from other Parkinson's patients who have used mucuna. Join online forums and communities. Get involved. Members often share valuable information about their experiences with different supplements.

5. Batch-to-batch variability. They can vary in levodopa concentration, which affects their effectiveness. Standardized products guarantee results.

6. Reputable retailers. Avoid unreliable sellers and independent seller platforms. Buy directly from the manufacturer's website or from certified pharmacies. Choose products that offer an authenticity code.

7. Shipping. Check that the quality of the product is maintained during transport, without exposure to extreme temperatures. Return the product if it does not meet your expectations or arrives damaged.

8. Keep a health journal after starting mucuna. Document your symptoms and any side effects. This record will be very valuable during your appointments with your doctor.

9. Reliable laboratories. In Europe and the United States, they are generally reliable regarding the safety of the product. However, sometimes the actual content does not match what is advertised. Stay alert.

10. Seed powders vs. extracts. Seed powders often lack precise information on content (cannot be guaranteed as it depends on plant conditions), it will range from 3% to 6% levodopa. Extracts should come with a certificate, but the actual levodopa content may differ from what is stated on the label.

11. Demand a certificate of analysis. You have the right to make sure you are getting what you pay for.

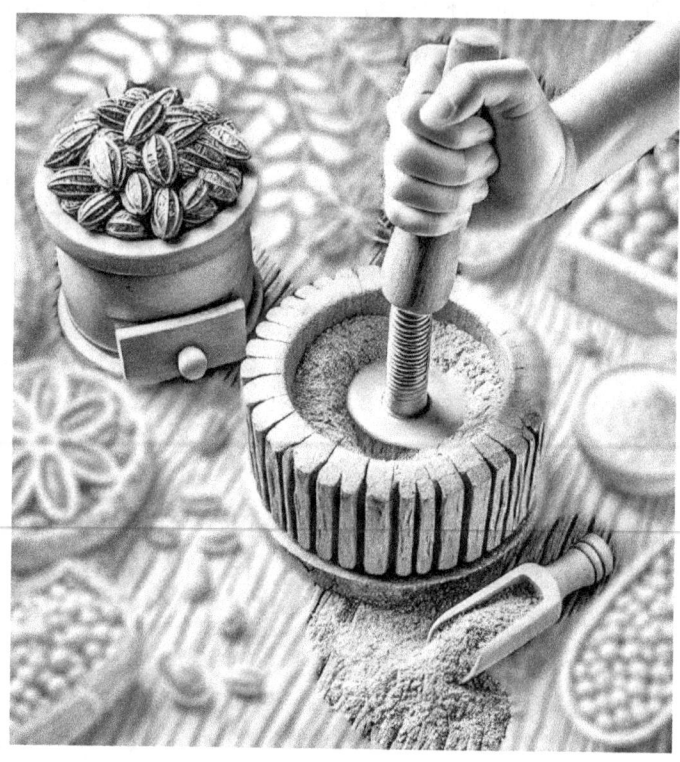

FIGURE 4. STANDARDIZED PURE POWDER

Several laboratories follow the traditional method: simply drying and grinding the mucuna seeds (sometimes other parts of the plant). A pure mucuna powder is obtained, approved but without artificial extracts. The percentage of levodopa cannot be assured, as it depends on the harvest, but an average of 4% (between 2.5 and 6.5%) is estimated.

4. Pure seeds or whole plant powder

Mucuna pruriens (MP) has been used for centuries in traditional medicine for its multiple health benefits. It is notable for its levodopa content (precursor of dopamine) but also contains other bioactive compounds that offer antioxidant, neuroprotective and adaptogenic effects.

It can be consumed in several forms, each with its specific characteristics and applications: seed powder, stem and leaf powder, extracts (liquid and powder) and variations of these extracts.

PURE MUCUNA SEEDS POWDER

Mucuna pruriens seed powder is the most common and traditional way of consuming this plant. It is obtained by drying and grinding the seeds into a fine powder. This powder is rich in levodopa, generally containing between 3% and 7% levodopa although the concentration may be higher in standardized products.

Due to its high levodopa content, seed powder is effective for Parkinson's motor symptoms such as rigidity and tremor. It is also adaptogenic and improves mood, reduces stress and increases sexual vitality (traditionally, it increases libido and is used in erectile dysfunction).

The pure powder obtained from the seeds can be consumed directly mixed with water, juices or in smoothies.

PURE POWDER CAPSULES

This powder obtained directly from the crushed seeds is also encapsulated to facilitate dosing and consumption. These capsules obviously have a lower proportion of levodopa than those of extracts, and this confuses many consumers, so attention must be paid to the content.

MUCUNA STEMS AND LEAVES POWDER

Mucuna pruriens stem and leaf powder is less common than the seed powder, but is still valued in traditional medicine, especially in Ayurvedic therapy. This powder is made by drying and grinding the aerial parts of the plant (stems and leaves), which contain a lower concentration of levodopa, but are rich in compounds such as flavonoids, saponins and tannins. They have different uses.

The stem and leaf powder are rich in antioxidants, which helps fight oxidative stress and inflammation. The compounds present in the stems and leaves can help strengthen the immune system and improve the body overall resistance.

INFUSIONS and DECOCTIONS of this powdered whole plant are drunk to relieve various disorders and are usually mixed with other herbal remedies.

LEVODOPA PERCENTAGE

The concentration of levodopa in seed powder or other unprocessed plant parts can vary significantly depending on several factors, such as:

- Plant variety: different varieties of Mucuna pruriens have different chemical profiles.

- Growing conditions: climate, soil and agricultural practices influence the levodopa content.

- Seed maturity: The concentration of levodopa may vary depending on the degree of maturity of the seed at the time of harvest.

- Drying and roasting process: these stages can affect the stability of levodopa and other compounds.

CONCENTRATIONS RANGE

Although it is difficult to establish an exact value, it is estimated that unprocessed mucuna seed powder can range from 1.25% to 9.16% levodopa, but the usual concentration of levodopa is between 3 and 7% of the dry weight of the seeds. This means that for every 100 grams of powder, there are usually between 3 and 7 grams (3,000 to 7,000 mg levodopa).

Weather changes during plant growth, soil type and

time of harvest, laboratories do not dare to give a percentage of levodopa, and this is understandable.

For practical purposes and as far as simple seed powder is concerned and focusing on the moment just after the grinding, but without taking extractions into account, we can consider that it will contain 4% levodopa unless the brand certifies otherwise: 4 grams out of every hundred are 4000 mg of levodopa in 100 grams, 400 mg every 10 grams, 200 mg every 5 grams.

Therefore, in most of these powdered mucuna seed products, an average teaspoon (5 milliliters capacity, 3 grams weight) contains between 150 and 250 milligrams of levodopa in case they contain what they say, in other words between 1½ Sinemet Plus tablets (150 mg LD) and one Sinemet 25/250 tablet (250 mg LD), but be careful because its clinical effect is four times lower (if carbidopa is not added) and that the side effects are also lower.

BIOAVAILABILITY, DOSAGE

Bioavailability: levodopa in raw powder may have lower bioavailability compared to concentrated and standardized extracts. This is due to the presence of other compounds in the seed that may interfere with absorption.

- Dosage: Due to the variability in levodopa concentration, it is difficult to establish a precise dosage for the unprocessed powder. This may increase the risk of overdose or suboptimal efficacy.

- Purity: unprocessed powder may contain impurities such as fibers, starch and other plant compounds, which can affect the quality of the product.

DO NOT DOSE WITH SPOONS

In the information sheets I provide about mucuna powder, I have estimated that a standard teaspoon (tsp) contains approximately 3 grams of powder. This measurement is only a comparative reference but is not exact nor recommended for precise dosing.

The problem with teaspoons is that they vary widely in size and capacity. Although they are generally assumed to have a capacity of 5 milliliters, not all teaspoons found at home match this measurement. Also, while 5 milliliters of water weigh 5 grams, the weight of powders varies depending on their density and texture. For example, in the case of flour, a level teaspoon usually weighs 3 grams, but if the teaspoon is heaped, it can weigh up to 5 grams. However, how heaped does it have to be for accuracy?

To facilitate comparisons, I have used the weight of 3 grams of flour in a level teaspoon as a reference in the sheets, since it is the most similar in density to mucuna powder. Some brands, such as Zandopa, provide 12-milliliter measuring cups to measure 7.5 grams, which indicates that approximately 5 milliliters of this powder could be equivalent to 3 grams in a teaspoon.

However, not all brands are consistent in their measuring utensils. Some include much smaller measuring cups, such as those that only measure 1/8 tsp (approximately 0.625 grams). This makes relying on teaspoons to measure precise doses quite risky, especially when dealing with highly concentrated powders.

For example, if you need to take 50 or 100 mg of levodopa and you have a powder that is 99% concentrated, how could you accurately measure it using a teaspoon or even a household scale? Household scales often do not have the sensitivity to accurately measure such small amounts.

My recommendation is to opt for products with lower concentrations to make dosing easier. If you need higher doses with ultra-concentrated products, it is safest to buy them in pre-measured capsules, which guarantees greater precision and safety in their use.

PURE SEED POWDER BRANDS

Here, we will discuss the most popular brands of laboratories that market simple mucuna seed powder, without extracting its components.

They are sold in bags and the patient must measure them by weighing them on precision scales, using the measuring cup provided, or with a teaspoon which is supposed to be equivalent to 5 milliliters (about 3 grams of weight for this type of powder).

There are many variations in its volume and this method is imprecise, but this teaspoon (*tsp* as used in British abbreviation) will allow us to give an average measurement to compare the approximate content of levodopa between brands. Above all, compared mostly to other non-pure powders, at high extraction power (up to 99%), we will see the enormous differences with this simple pure powder.

ZANDOPA powder - *zanducare.com*

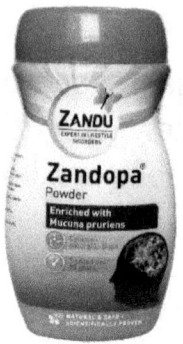
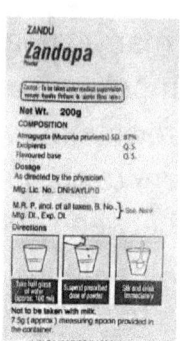

PURE POWDER	3.3 %	1 tsp = **100 mg** LD
seeds	3 grams	

Zandopa is the reference mucuna in the trials conducted with patients (HP-200) and was standardized so that each 7.5 gram *vial (which comes with a container) contains 250 mg of levodopa. That represents 3.3%, so a teaspoon (3 grams) would contain 100 mg of LD.

The powder comes directly from seeds but is standardized to ensure quality. Since it is not an extract, you have to take more quantity, and some patients complain about its taste.

---

*In an external analysis of several brands, the percentage of levodopa in Zandopa was even higher than advertised: 357 mg in 7.5 grams (4.7%).

BULKSUPPLEMENTS powder -
bulksupplements.com

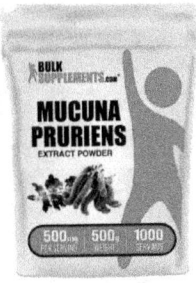 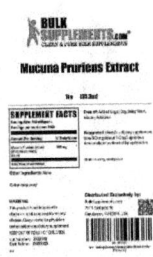

PURE POWDER	4 %	1 tsp = **120 mg** LD
seeds	3 grams	

BulkSupplements offers bulk supplements, which makes them more affordable. They are known for their high purity, no additives, and they include Mucuna pruriens. They sent me a certificate of analysis, but as it is usual with seed powder, they do not give a percentage of levodopa and we will calculate it at an average of 4%.

In these presentations, the taste can be unpleasant, and attention must be paid to precise dosage, which requires knowledge and the appropriate tools.

CARMEL Organics powder - *bulksupplements.com*

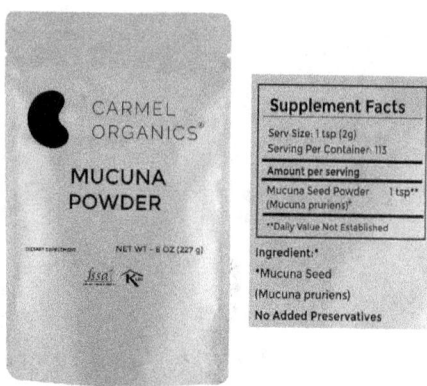

PURE POWDER	4 %	1 tsp = **120 mg** LD
seeds	3 grams	

Carmel Organics was founded in 2012 and is focused on supporting small farmers in India through organic cultivation of herbs and spices.

Pure seed powder that, like the vast majority, cannot guarantee the percentage of levodopa that ranges between 2.5 and 6, and which we estimate for simplicity at an average of 4% unless the manufacturer indicates otherwise.

They recommend a dose of half a teaspoon, which they equate to 2 grams. Given the variable capacity of teaspoons, we are considering 3 grams of the product here to balance potency comparisons between brands.

NOVA NUTRITIONS powder- *bulksupplements.com*

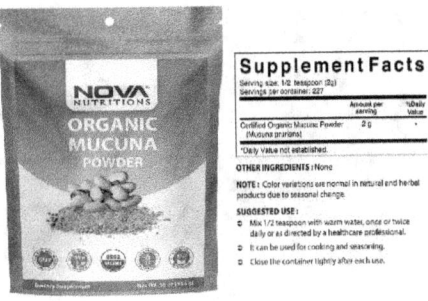

PURE POWDER	4 %	1 tsp = **120 mg** LD
seeds	*3 grams*	

Pure seed powder. They cannot guarantee the percentage of levodopa, which ranges between 2.5 and 6. For simplicity, we estimate an average of 4% of levodopa unless the manufacturer indicates otherwise.

They recommend a dose of half a teaspoon, which they equate to 2 grams. Given the variable capacity of teaspoons, we are considering 3 grams of the product here to balance potency comparisons between brands.

NUTRICOST powder - *nutricost.com*

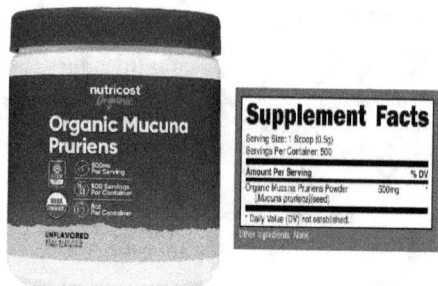

PURE POWDER	4 %	1 tsp = **120 mg** LD
seeds	3 grams	

Pure seed powder as long as they do not mention it as an extract. In these products we estimate an average of 4% of levodopa. That is 120 mg of levodopa for an average teaspoon (3 grams).

They recommend a low dose, a half-gram vial, which would represent only 20 mg of levodopa. This way, it can be considered a dietary supplement instead of a medicine, and some bureaucratic hurdles are avoided. In patients, the ration or dose does not depend on the manufacturer but on the doctor.

KAPIKACCHU powder - *banyambotanicals.com*

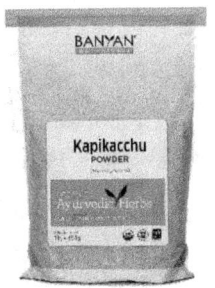
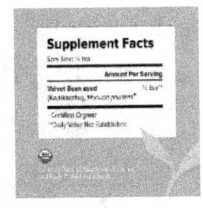

PURE POWDER	4.5 %	1 tsp = **135 mg** LD
seeds	3 grams	

They have sent me a Certificate of Analysis and they explain that their seed powder, depending on the growing conditions, has a levodopa percentage between 4 and 5%. Taking the average of 4.5%, a teaspoon (3 grams) is equivalent to 135 mg of levodopa.

HERBS FOREVER powder - *herbsforever.com*

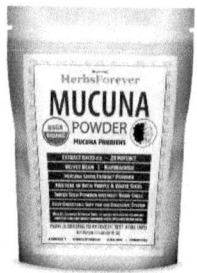 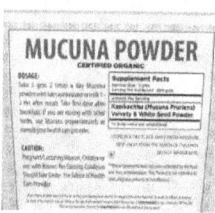

PURE POWDER	4.75 %	1 tsp = **142 mg** LD
seeds	3 grams	

I wrote to the laboratory to clarify the concentration of levodopa, and they replied that, although in mucuna powder it usually varies between 2 and 5%, their product contains between 3.5 and 6%.

I have considered the average of 4.75% to obtain the result of 142.5 mg of levodopa in each teaspoon (3 grams).

PURE POWDER IN CAPSULES OR TABLETS

In other laboratories, the pure powder (without extractions) is encapsulated to avoid the taste that some find unpleasant. The problem is that the amount of levodopa is low unless the capsule is large (difficult to swallow) or the "serving" includes several capsules.

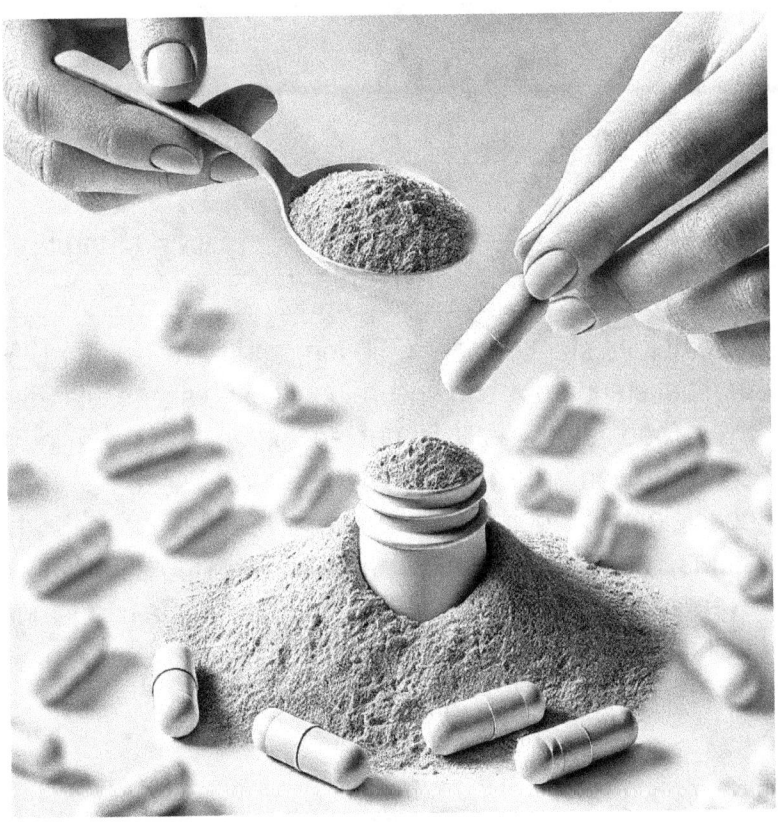

HIMALAYA organic - *iherbs.com*

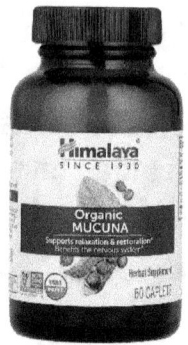
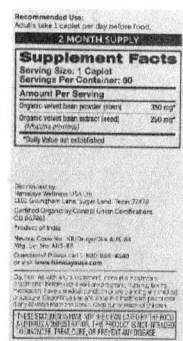

Capsule PURE POWDER	0.25 and 4 %	1 caps = **11 mg** LD
stem and seeds	*600 mg*	

It combines stem powder (350 mg) and seed powder (250 mg) but standardized to ensure quality and encapsulated to avoid bad taste. As it is not an extract, it has a lower concentration of levodopa. The 250 mg of seeds at 4% is equivalent to 10 mg LD. There is less levodopa in the stems, between 0.19-0.31%) and taking 0.25% as an average, the 350 mg is only 1.4 mg of levodopa (but it must include other active substances).

SWANSON capsules powder – *swansoneurope.com*

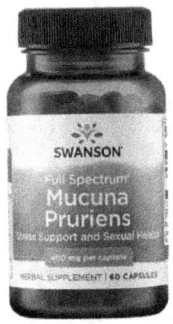
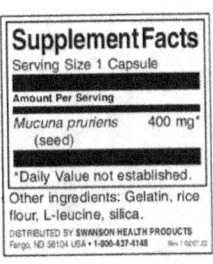

Capsule PURE POWDER	4 %	1 caps = **16 mg** LD
seeds	400 mg	

To avoid the bad taste of the seed powder, it has been encapsulated. It is 400 mg of the ground, without making any extract, which has been wrapped. As it is not an extract, it has a lower concentration of levodopa, and you have to take more for the same dose.

It contains little levodopa, like seed powders, and usually varies between 2 and 7%. If we take 4% as an average, each capsule contains 14 mg of levodopa.

SUPREME capsules powder – *supremenaturals.com*

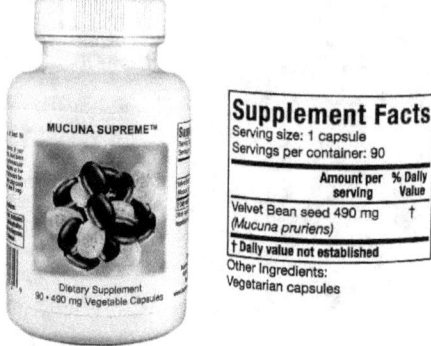

Capsule PURE POWDER	4 %	
seeds	490 mg	1 capsule = **20 mg** LD

Another option is to take mucuna seeds simply ground, without extracts or other artificial additives: 490 mg of raw seed powder, whose percentage of levodopa varies between 2 and 7%. If we take 4% as an average, each capsule contains 22 mg of levodopa.

Useful if you want to start using mucuna without risks, and later, you would have to take several capsules per dose : with 5 you would have 110 mg, a little more than the levodopa that Sinemet 25/100 has, adjusting the clinical potency due to the lack of carbidopa .

BANYAN tablets - *banyanbotanicals.com*

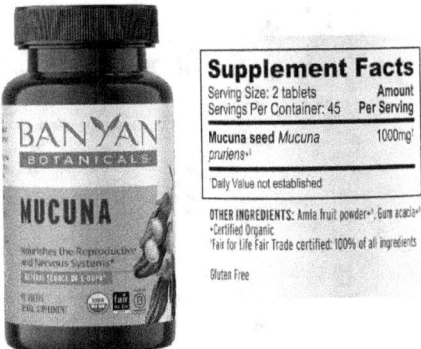

PURE POWDER Tablet	4.5 %	1 caps = **22 mg** LD
seeds	500 mg	

Now in tablets, pure seeds in powder, according to traditional principles in this laboratory.

It's like taking Zandopa, but packaged, so that the taste is not an impediment. According to the quality certification of their product, it ensures 4.5% of levodopa. Each tablet would only have approximately 22.5 mg, of course with all the components of the seeds, but without any other processed ingredients.

BRIEOFOOD capsules powder – *brieofood.com*

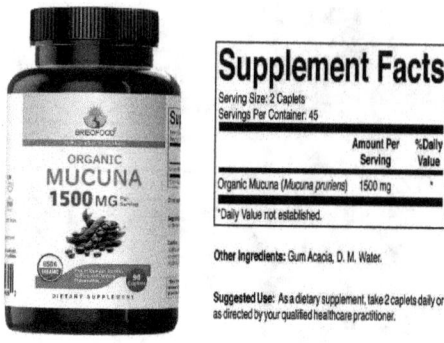

PURE POWDER Tablet	4 %	1 tablet = **30 mg** LD
seeds	750 mg	

It is among the tablets or capsules that contain the largest amount of pure seed powder, simply ground, without extracts or other artificial additives: 750 mg of raw seed powder, whose percentage of levodopa varies between 2 and 7%. If we take 4% as an average, each capsule contains 30 mg of levodopa. With normal doses, 2 or more are needed.

The capsule is relatively large for a low amount of levodopa, but it ensures purity, without additives, and avoids the peculiar taste of the powder.

61

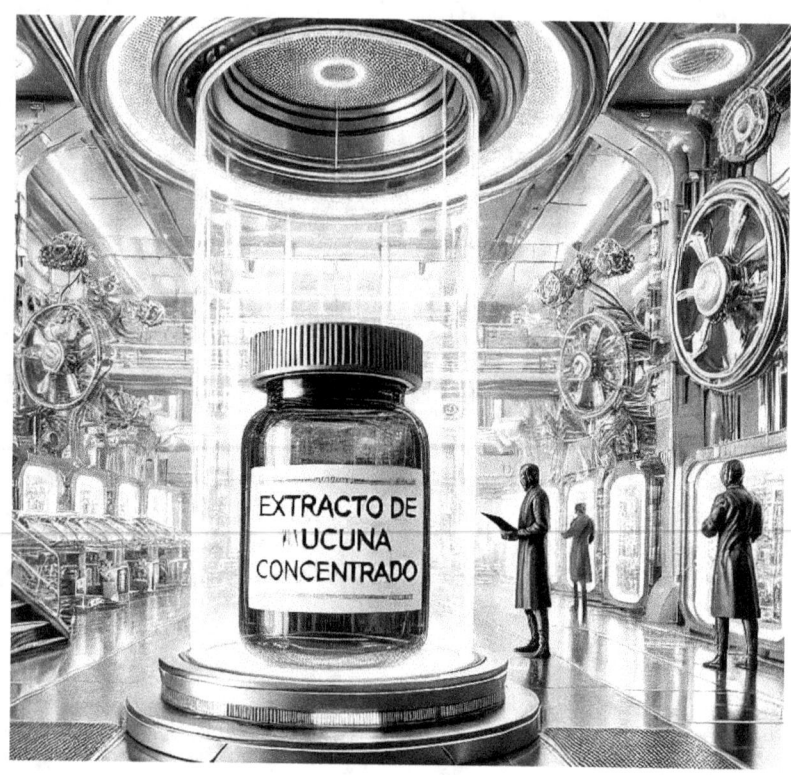

FIGURE 5. CONCENTRATED MUCUNA EXTRACTS. The process is more complicated and concentrated extracts of the plant are obtained, with levodopa percentages between 15 and 99%.

5. Low-concentrated extracts

Concentrated extracts of mucuna seeds, or of the entire plant, have gained popularity due to their potential therapeutic benefits. Throughout the manufacturing process, the aim is to obtain extracts that maximize both levodopa and other bioactive compounds that make this plant an interesting natural alternative.

THE PROCEDURE

It includes plant selection and drying, grinding, component extraction, filtration and concentration, standardization, encapsulation or formulation, and quality control.

1. Selection and drying

It all starts with a very careful selection of the Mucuna pruriens seeds. The best ones are chosen, ensuring that they are ripe and free of impurities.

The seeds are then dried at a low temperature to protect the active compounds, especially levodopa, which is sensitive to heat. In some cases, they are lightly roasted, which can help improve the body ability to absorb these compounds.

2. Fine grinding

Once dried, the seeds are ground into a very fine powder. This is important because it facilitates the extraction of active compounds such as levodopa. A fine powder offers more surface area during the extraction process, thus maximizing efficiency.

3. Extraction of bioactive components

Extraction is the heart of the process. There are several techniques to extract as much levodopa and other compounds as possible:

- Solvent selection: Depending on the compounds to be extracted, solvents such as water, ethanol or methanol are used. This also depends on the regulations that control solvent residues in the final product.

- Extraction techniques such as

- Maceration or infusion: the seed powder is immersed in a solvent for a long time, allowing soluble compounds, such as levodopa, to dissolve.

- Reflux extraction: here the solvent is heated and circulated through the powder, which increases the efficiency of the process.

- Supercritical CO_2 extraction: this is a more advanced and cleaner technique that uses carbon dioxide in a special state, allowing for obtaining high purity extracts.

- Ultrasound or Microwave: modern methods that accelerate the extraction process without damaging the active compounds.

4. Filtration and concentration

The liquid obtained from the extraction goes through a filtration process to separate the extract from the solid residues. This liquid extract is then concentrated, removing excess solvent. This can be done by vacuum evaporation to avoid the use of high temperatures that could degrade the active compounds.

5. Standardization (Normalization)

This step is crucial to ensure that the final extract has a uniform concentration of levodopa. The content is analysed and, if necessary, adjusted to ensure that it meets the required standards (e.g. a minimum concentration of 15% levodopa).

6. Encapsulation or formulation

Once the concentrated extract is obtained, it can be encapsulated or prepared into other forms, such as tablets or liquids.

This step also involves packaging under controlled conditions to protect the product from light, air and moisture, ensuring its stability and efficacy.

7. Quality Control

Quality control ensures that the final product is safe and effective. Tests are performed to confirm the concentration of levodopa and the absence of contaminants and to verify that the product is stable during storage.

TYPES OF EXTRACTS

There are different presentations of extracts, each with its own advantages and characteristics, depending on the user's needs.

Mucuna liquid extracts

Liquid extracts of Mucuna pruriens concentrate the active ingredients in a solution. These extracts are known to be more potent and act faster than powdered extracts. Typically, the concentration of levodopa in these products is standardized at 15% or more, ensuring effective dosing.

Given their high bioavailability (they are rapidly absorbed into the body), liquid extracts are ideal for treating Parkinson's motor symptoms immediately. In addition to levodopa, they contain other compounds that may have neuroprotective effects and improve cognitive function.

They are usually administered in drops under the tongue or diluted in water, which facilitates rapid absorption.

Mucuna extracts powder

Powdered extracts are another very popular format. They are obtained by evaporating the solvent used in the extraction, resulting in a fine, concentrated powder. These extracts can have a levodopa concentration ranging from 15% to 30%, making them much more potent than simple seed powder.

Powdered extracts are especially useful for those who need medium or high doses of levodopa. It is crucial to follow the recommended dosages, as these are concentrated products, and incorrect use could cause unwanted side effects.

Standard and complex extracts

Standard seed-based extracts are formulated to contain a precise amount of levodopa, making them ideal for medical treatments where consistency is key. These extracts allow for more exact dosage control, which is vital in the management of Parkinson's.

On the other hand, complex extracts offer a more varied mix of plant compounds, not just levodopa. This is interesting when looking for a more synergistic effect, taking advantage of other beneficial compounds such as antioxidants, flavonoids and saponins, which can enhance the overall effect of the treatment.

Ultra-concentrated extracts

Some patients seek out extremely concentrated extracts, which promise up to 99% levodopa. However, these products are not always the best option. This high level of concentration is achieved through artificial procedures that, although effective, eliminate many of the natural components that make Mucuna pruriens a special alternative.

Additionally, there can be issues with dosing. For example, if you buy a powder with 99% levodopa, how do you correctly calculate a small dose like 50 or 100 milligrams? Sometimes labels are inaccurate or do not offer reliable concentration certificates, which adds a level of uncertainty. Ultra-concentrated extracts may be useful in very specific cases, but I do not recommend them for general use.

It is always better to opt for more balanced extracts, which retain a portion of the additional compounds that improve the bioavailability of levodopa.

Extracts in capsules: convenience and precision

A practical option is those containing between 15% and 40% levodopa. These products are easier to dose and offer the advantage of maintaining a large part of the plant natural compounds. As treatment progresses, and if the patient needs more levodopa, the use of more potent extracts (50% or more) may be considered, always under medical supervision.

When evaluating capsules, it is important to look at how many milligrams of extract each contains, not just the percentage of levodopa. Some capsules may have a lower concentration of levodopa but make up for it with a higher amount of extract, which can make them just as effective.

CHOOSING THE RIGHT PRODUCT

Depending on the therapeutic objective, it is essential to choose the appropriate format of Mucuna pruriens:

- Seed powder: ideal if you are looking for a more natural and less processed product, with a focus on Parkinson's treatment and general well-being.

- Stem and leaf powder: this format offers antioxidant and anti-inflammatory benefits although it is not as specific for Parkinson's.

- Liquid and powder extracts: recommended for those who need high doses of levodopa, such as in advanced Parkinson's, or for those seeking to improve their physical or cognitive performance.

Ultra-concentrated extracts : due to their potency, they are difficult to dose and should be used with great caution, preferably in capsules.

CHOOSING THE RIGHT DOCTOR

Mucuna is sold freely, but the treatment must be supervised by a doctor. And choosing a doctor is more important than buying the product. He must know Parkinson's disease well, as well as mucuna so that he can calculate the doses. He must be a good communicator, able to show empathy with you, and to talk freely about your symptoms, your improvements or the adverse effects, without any reservations and without fear of being reproached too much, even for spontaneous decisions that you make and that may have harmed you.

RANGE OF THERAPEUTIC APPLICATIONS

Mucuna pruriens offers a wide range of therapeutic applications, from natural extracts to highly concentrated formulations. Choosing the right product depends on each person's needs, and the precise treatment will be tailored to their individual levodopa metabolization profile, their age, the clinical form and the evolutionary phase of their disease. It is also important to balance the amount of levodopa and bioactive compounds to obtain the best results.

MOST POPULAR BRANDS

Below we will discuss the main brands of concentrated seed extracts in capsules. We have ordered them from the lowest to highest concentration. The least concentrated ones will have a lower percentage of levodopa, but they are more like the original plant. An excessive extraction, some do it at 90-99%, has more levodopa, but other constituents of mucuna which are important for its best functioning will be missing. If the levodopa is at 99%, practically none of the components that make mucuna special will remain. Whatever little or large concentration they have, you must evaluate how many grams of extract they contain. There are brands at 15% but with larger capsules making them contain in the end more levodopa.

Moreover, you must not pay attention to the dosage recommended by the laboratory because it must be prescribed by the doctor, and they are misleading when they give the figures for levodopa "per serving", which can be 2 capsules and sometimes more.

We will focus on the most common product extracts at 15-25%. Among those of the same concentration, I will order them from the lowest to highest amount of levodopa, namely from the least one, being the 10- mg capsule of Pure Encapsulations to the most being the 171-mg capsule of Herbs Forever. Let us also mention a curious gummy extract product with a very low percentage of levodopa (5%).

ETTA VITA - *ettavita.com*

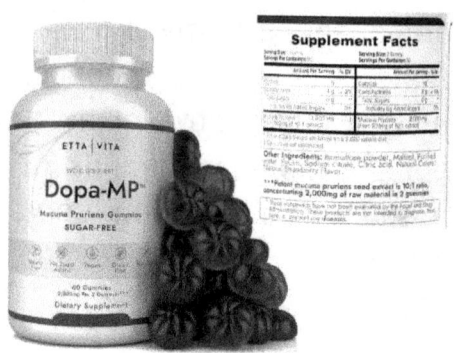

Gummy EXTRACT	5 %	1 rubber = **5 mg** LD
seeds	100 mg	

Interesting mucuna extract in GUMMIES, which are absorbed in part under the tongue (Dopa-MP gummies). In theory, it is useful for those who have problems with gastric emptying, which slows down absorption and causes a drop in appetite after eating. But in a small amount of levodopa.

Each gummy contains 100 mg of seeds, 10:1 extract. According to the laboratory, it is estimated that there is 5% levodopa, and in each gummy (100 mg) there are 5 mg of levodopa. It is very little, but it opens the way to the sublingual route.

PURE ENCAPSULATIONS - *pureencapsulations.com*

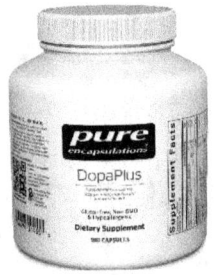

Capsule EXTRACT	15 %	1 capsule = 10 **mg** LD
seeds + B6 + tea	66 mg	

The serving is 200 mg of 15% seed extract (30 mg total) but it is distributed in 3 capsules: each one containing only 66 mg, or 10 mg of levodopa.

Added with green tea extract (33 mg with 70% catecholamine EGCG = 23 mg), B6 (2.2 mg) and others in insignificant quantities.

ADVANCE PHYSICIAN - *physicianformulas.com*

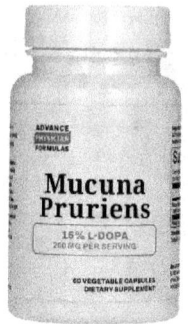 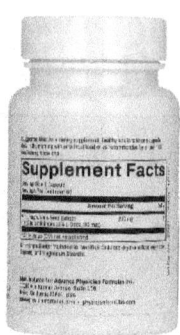

Capsule EXTRACT	15 %	1 capsule = 30 **mg** LD
seeds	200 mg	

It is a brand with good products, but it falls short with mucuna. The low content of levodopa (30 mg per capsule) is justified because an extract has been sought that minimizes the risks of overdose.

The risk is certainly low, since in a publication (Soumyanath A et al 2018) these capsules were analyzed and only contained 12 mg of levodopa, 40% of the advertised information.

SOLARAY Dopabean – *solaray.com*

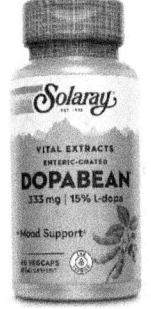
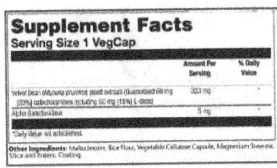

Capsule EXTRACT	15 %	1 caps = **50 mg** LD
seeds	*333 mg*	

Seed extract containing one-fifth of catecholamines, of which at least 50 mg (15%) is levodopa.

According to a scientific study (Soumyanath A et al 2018) that analyzed the capsules, something more was targeted: 56 mg of levodopa per capsule. It is one of the brands in which an external analysis verifies that they contain what they advertise. On Amazon.com it is a selected option.

HORBÄACH - *pipingrock.com*

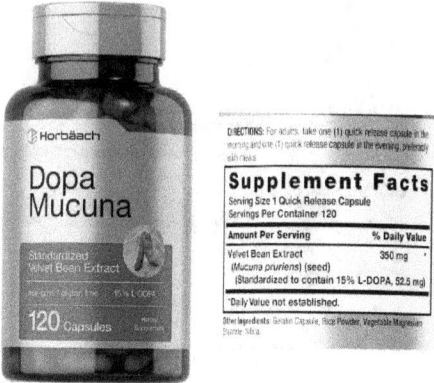

Capsule EXTRACT	15 %	1 caps = **52 mg** LD
seeds	350 mg	

15% extract, a moderate concentration that allows 52.5 mg of levodopa in a small, rapid-release capsule (350 mg of product).

PIPING ROCK - *pipingrock.com*

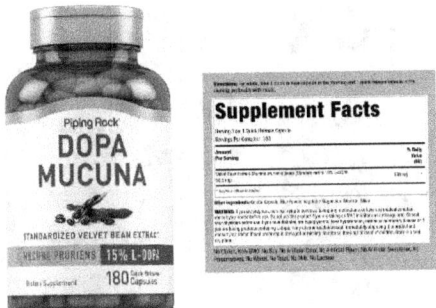

Capsule EXTRACT	15 %	1 caps = **52 mg** LD
seeds	350 mg	

Rapid release capsules of a 15% extract using water and alcohol, which they detail in their response, along with several certificates of analysis.

DOPA MUCUNA NOW - *nowfoods.com*

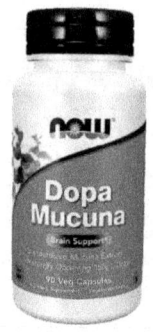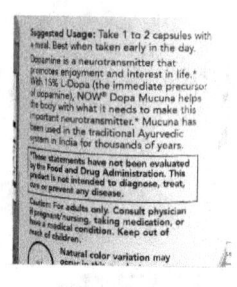

Capsule EXTRACT	15 %	1 caps = **60 mg** LD
seeds	400 mg	

It is a prestigious brand, selected on *Amazon.com* with ratings of more than 4/5 stars, frequent purchases and few returns.

Good ratio between the low potency of the extract and the levodopa content, 60 mg, in an acceptable-sized capsule (400 mg).

The label shows 800 mg (120 of levodopa) because the recommended "serving" is two capsules.

BONUSAN mucuna – *bonusan.com*

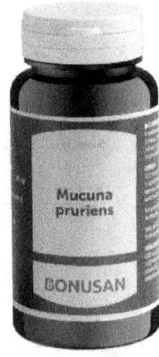
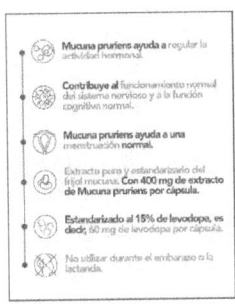

Capsule EXTRACT	15 %	1 capsule = **60 mg** LD
seeds	400 mg	

Another good brand, practically the same as the previous one, with a 15% seed extract, one of the most used.

Bonusan had been able to maintain production when there were supply problems to obtain other brands of mucuna.

DOUBLE WOOD - *doublewood.com*

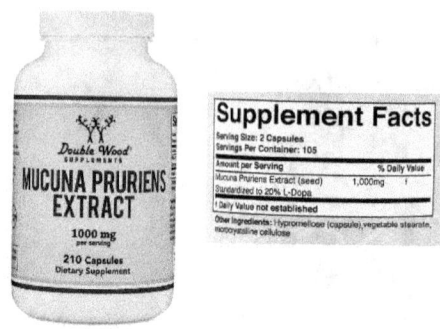

Capsule EXTRACT	20 %	1 caps = **100 mg** LD
seeds	500 mg	

Again, it should be noted that the serving (1000 mg) is two capsules: each one contains 500 mg of 20% seed extract, that is, 100 mg of natural levodopa, one of the highest amounts for low concentration extracts.

ZAZZEE - *zazzeenaturals.com*

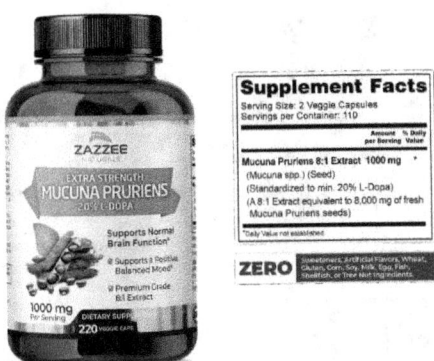

Capsule EXTRACT	20 %	1 caps = **100 mg** LD
seeds	500 mg	

They advertise that the serving is 1000 mg distributed in two capsules. Each capsule contains 500 mg of 20% seed extract, or 100 mg of natural levodopa. That is rather much for a low concentration extract.

KETER Wellness - *keterwellness.com*

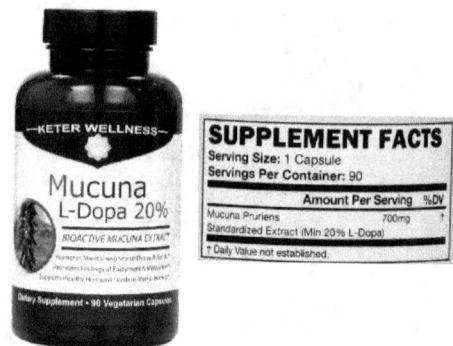

Capsule EXTRACT	20 %	1 caps = **140 mg** LD
seeds	700 mg	

The capsule must be large because it contains 700 mg, and the highest levodopa content (140 mg) is found in low concentration extracts (20%).

For those who want high potency levodopa without overly strong extracts, it is an option, but not everyone can swallow capsules of that size.

VITAKRUID – *vitakruid.nl*

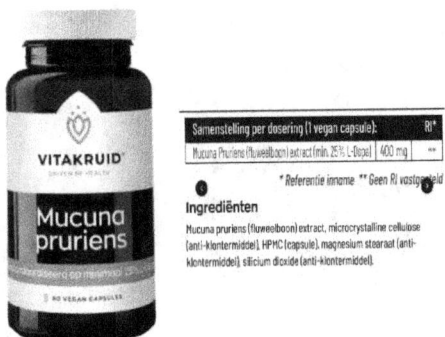

Capsule EXTRACT	25 %	1 caps = **100 mg** LD
seeds	*400 mg*	

It is a Dutch brand that is widely consumed in the country. The 25% is a concentration in the high to moderate range, which allows for 100 mg of levodopa in 400 mg of product.

This makes the capsule relatively small for that amount of active substance.

MACUDOPA - *macudopausa.com*

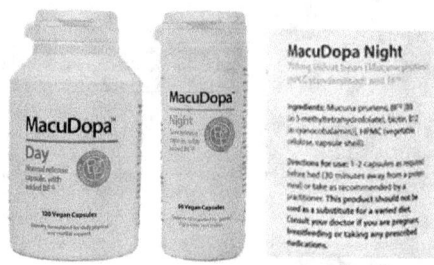

Capsule EXTRACT	15 %	1 capsule = **100 mg** LD
day and night	700 mg	

An interesting option with a 700-mg extract (it does not clarify whether from seeds or the whole plant) that standardizes for 100 mg of levodopa (15% deducted). They differentiate the night capsule that they advertise as delayed release. This "delayed" night-time mucuna, if it really is, could be an important option regarding patients with dyskinesias given in the daytime; its slow action would be reminiscent of Sinemet Retard or Madopar HBS, but with the advantage of using natural levodopa. Let's mention minimal amounts of vitamins B7, B9 and B12, which are not relevant.

HERBSFOREVER - *herbsforever.com*

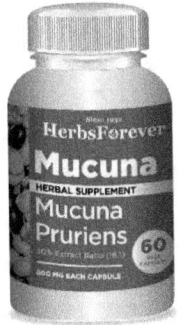 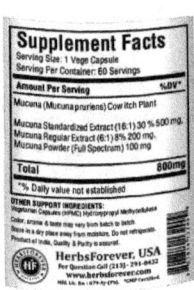

Capsule EXTRACT	30, 8 and 5 %	1 caps = **171 mg** LD
seeds	800 mg	

It is an interesting combination of seed extracts of different potencies: 500 mg at 30% (150 mg LD), 200 mg at 8% and 100 mg at 5%. This gives an average extraction of 21.375% with 171 mg of levodopa.

At least in theory, it allows levodopa potency while maintaining other constituents. Their response is detailed and they are open to customizing their products. In one publication (Soumyanath A et al 2018), another product of theirs had less levodopa than advertised, but it has since been withdrawn from the market.

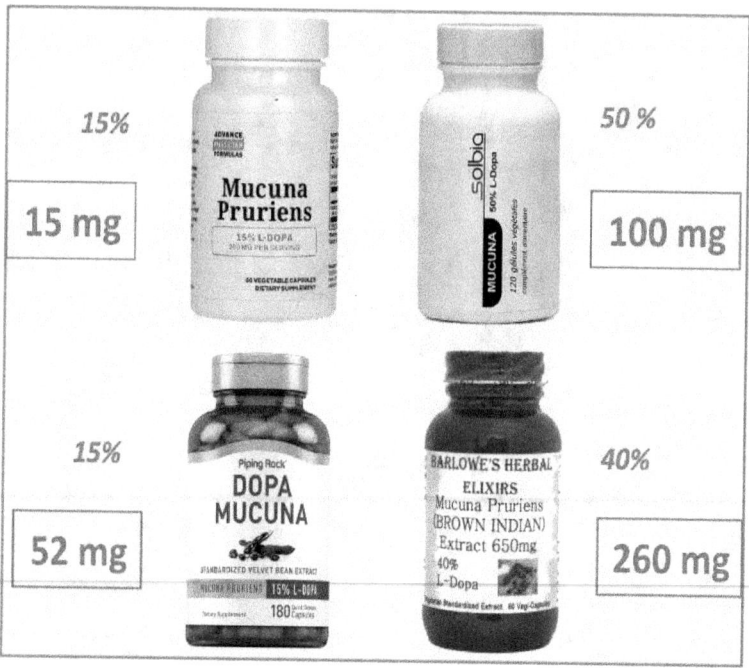

FIGURE 6. CONTENT AND PERCENTAGES

In extracts, we must differentiate between the potency and concentration of levodopa because the amount of mucuna influences this. We see two at 15% with large differences per capsule: 15 and 52 mg. And a 50% extract of 100 mg, less than half of the 40% (260 mg).

The content, method of extraction and percentage of levodopa influence the size of the capsule.

6. Medium-concentrated extracts (40-60%)

Medium strength extracts (40-60% levodopa) are the most popular. It is appealing that about half of the content is levodopa and this suggests, in principle, that it will be more effective and in a smaller capsule.

When the patient needs to increase the daily levodopa, having small capsules with enough levodopa is evidently important. It avoids the hassle of taking much powder that can be unpleasant in taste and cause flatulence or other abdominal discomfort.

At some point they will be necessary, but I do not recommend using them from the beginning, when a little simple seed powder may be enough, if necessary encapsulated to avoid bad taste or later capsules with low concentration extract (15-20%).

There are two main reasons. First, all extracts are made by artificial means, and the more concentrated they are, the more complex they are. Secondly, because the more levodopa they contain, the more substances in the plant that give them their special therapeutic efficacy have been wasted.

It is common sense to think that if mucuna seeds have 4% levodopa, the rest is a lot of substances that will be lost if it occupies half.

Therefore, I suggest that these extracts are reserved for later stages of development, when much more levodopa is needed.

On the other hand, with the guidelines that I will give later, by choosing to combine carbidopa or benserazide, the high doses of mucuna can be delayed even further.

BIOVEA - *biovea.com*

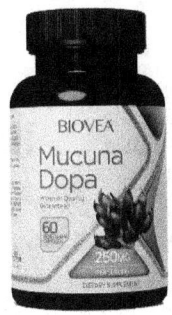

Capsule EXTRACT	40 %	1 caps = **100 mg** LD
seeds	*250 mg*	

It is a medium-grade extract (40%) and light weight (250 mg), which allows it to supply an acceptable amount of natural levodopa with a small volume capsule (easier to swallow): 100 mg (the same amount of synthetic levodopa that a Sinemet 25/100 contains).

We remember that in the absence of carbidopa, its efficacy on the symptoms would be equivalent to a quarter (like a quarter of Sinemet).

NUTRICOST - *nutricost.com*

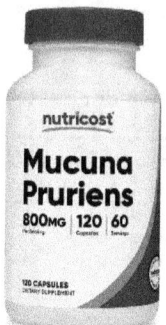
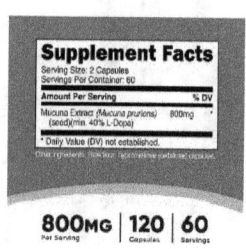

Capsule EXTRACT	40 %	
seeds	400 mg	1 caps = **160 mg** LD

The extract is of medium grade (40%) from a relatively large capsule (160 mg) which provides 160 mg of natural levodopa. That is slightly more than the levodopa in one and a half Sinemet Plus tablets, although without carbidopa its effectiveness for symptoms would be equivalent to 40 mg, less than half a Sinemet Plus or a quarter of a Madopar 50/200. It is a quality product, selected on amazon.com and with very good user ratings.

HEALTH Essentials - healthessentialsdirect.co.uk.com

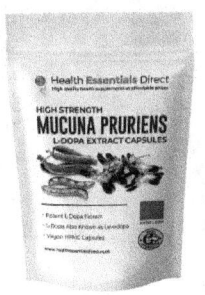
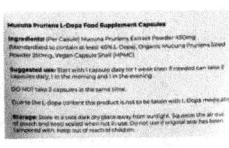

Capsule EXTRACT	40% + 4%	1 caps = **190 mg** LD
Seeds	700 mg	

An interesting product because, according to the label, it combines a (whole) plant extract standardized for levodopa at 40% (180 mg) and adds 250 mg of seeds (without extract) which, estimated at an average of 4%, would be another 10 mg of levodopa. That is, 190 mg of levodopa, most of which is from the whole plant.

It is one of the few products that extracts the entire plant, which allows it to preserve many of the unknown components of mucuna.

BARLOWE - *barloweherbalelixirs.com*

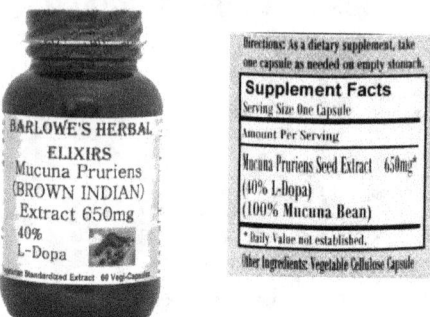

Capsule EXTRACT	40 %	1 capsule = **260 mg** LD
seeds	260 mg	

It is a very powerful product. The capsule is large and somewhat difficult to swallow (650 mg of extract), and with a concentration of 40%, it contains 260 mg of levodopa: more than a Sinemet 25/250 (blue) or a tablet and a quarter of Madopar.

If combined with carbidopa (either alone or by mixing part of Sinemet) it may be an excessive dose in a patient with a medium evolution. However, it is useful later, if a lot of levodopa is needed but one does not want to use ultra-concentrated levodopa.

SOLBIA – *en.solbia.com*

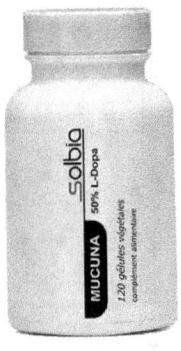

Capsule EXTRACT	50 %	1 caps = **100 mg** LD
seeds	*200 mg*	

Being a more concentrated extract than the previous ones (50%) it contains less levodopa because each capsule only contains 200 mg. It is the same levodopa in a Sinemet Plus tablet (or half a Madopar 50/200), and its theoretical clinical efficacy is 25 mg (a quarter of a Sinemet Plus) unless it is combined with this one: which would be almost equivalent. You have to be careful with the doses.

HERBAL POWERS MP – *herbal-powers.com*

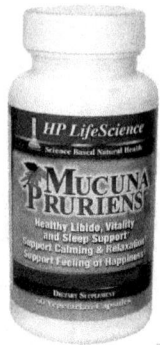
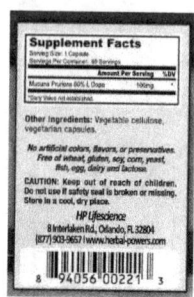

Capsule EXTRACT	60 %	1 caps = **60 mg** LD
seeds	100 mg	

It is only 100 mg of seed powder with an extract (60%), in the upper range of mid-grade ones. That would allow 60 mg in each small, easy-to-swallow capsule.

However, an external analysis (Soumyanath 2018) found amounts of levodopa much lower than advertised.

SOURCE NATURALS MDopa - *sourcenaturals.com*

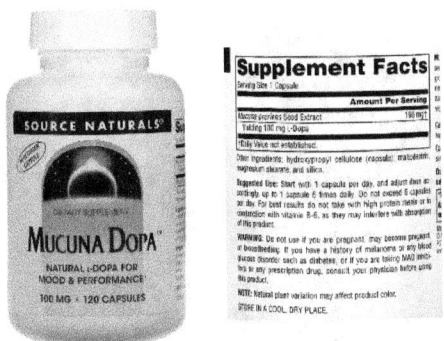

Capsule EXTRACT	60 %	1 caps = **100 mg** LD
seeds	166 mg	

The same option as above: a significant extract (60%) from a small amount of seeds (166 mg) leads to relatively small-sized capsules with an acceptable amount of levodopa: 100 mg.

According to an external analysis (Soumyanat 2018), it is even higher (120 mg of levodopa per capsule).

NUSAPURE - *nusapure.com*

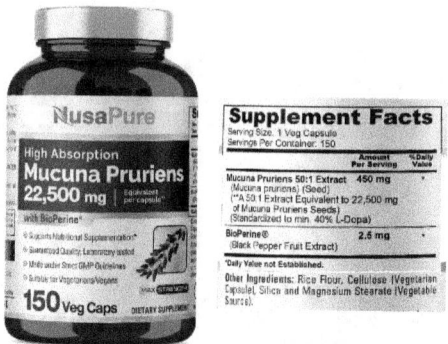

Capsule EXTRACT	40 %	1 caps = **180 mg** LD
seeds + piperine	450 mg	

Very interesting is the addition of BLACK PEPPER, which contains piperine, which seems to increase the absorption of levodopa (Hu 2024), and will be useful in patients with intestinal transit problems.

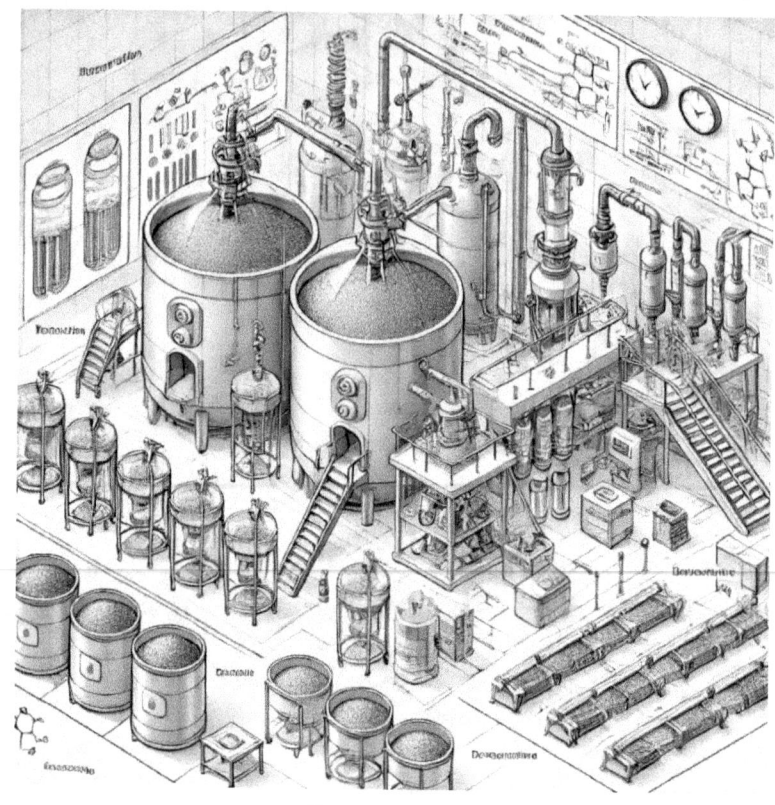

Ultra-concentrated extracts (more than 90% levodopa) require more complex and technologically advanced processes.

They are necessary in advanced cases, with strict medical supervision, but in previous phases patients may become confused if they use it in powder form, with the risk of overdose.

7. Ultra-concentrated extracts (>90%)

Very high concentration extracts (90% or more levodopa) are useful in advanced cases but difficult to manage in early or middle stages of the disease.

RISK OF OVERDOSE

They carry a high risk of overdose, especially in powder form. If you were to buy a packet of mucuna powder that is advertised as containing 99% levodopa, one teaspoon (3 grams) would consist of 3 grams of levodopa, in other words 3,000 milligrams, the same as 30 tablets of Sinemet 25/100 or 15 tablets of Madopar 50/200 provided it contains what it says.

Now, if you wanted to take the equivalent of one Sinemet Plus tablet, how would you dose the 100 mg you need from a spoonful of 3,000mg? Precision scales would be necessary in addition to a great deal of experience.

Imagine the risk for a person who is used to taking pure seed powder (4% levodopa) and who takes half a teaspoon (in Zandopa or similar) to receive 100 mg of levodopa. If he were to take half a teaspoon of the ultra-concentrated now, he would be taking 1500 mg (like 15 Sinemet Plus tablets).

Therefore, except for special cases of expert patients with good medical supervision, I do not recommend ultra-concentrated powder extracts.

Capsules can be used if you want to increase the levodopa level significantly. In advanced Parkinson's, an alternative is to use capsules with 99% powder, such as Clean Mucuna.

USEFUL IN ADVANCED CASES

It may be useful in the early stages of treatment for patients who insist on not taking carbidopa or any conventional drug. It is a way of improving symptoms, knowing that in order to obtain the efficacy of Sinemet Plus the dose of natural levodopa (which does not contain carbidopa or benserazide) must be multiplied by four.

But be careful if it is combined with Sinemet or Madopar tablets because their carbidopa or benserazide would also act on the levodopa in mucuna and may have undesirable effects.

CHEMICAL EXTRACTION METHODS

Another issue to bear in mind is that the chemical extraction process has been complex, and there is little that is natural left in what is sold.

WHAT IS LEFT OF THE PLANT?

Another major drawback of these ultra-concentrated extracts, whether you buy 99 % levodopa powder or capsules, is the minuscule 1% remaining. The other components of the plant, making it particularly suitable for treating Parkinson's disease, are lost.

OVERDOSE EUPHORIA

Some tell us wonders about these ultra-concentrated extracts insisting on the fact that it has given them a new life, that it works much better than others. They may be right; it works very well, but probably because they are over-medicated!

MICROINGREDIENTS – microingredients.com

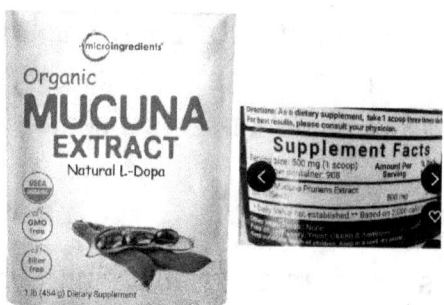

EXTRACT POWDER 20:1	% ?	1 tsp = **120 mg** LD?
seeds	cup, 250 mg?	

Incomplete information. The manufacturer's website and Amazon only state that the recommended serving is 500 mg of the product in 2 cups, the capacity of which is not mentioned. It is not pure powder, but an extract, and the proportion is not shown. It is a 20:1 ratio according to a photo provided by a customer.

It means that each part contains 20 times the weight of the plant; in other words, a teaspoon (3 grams) is equivalent to 6000 mg of seeds, and the usual 4% would be 120 milligrams of levodopa.

No email contact is given to request information.

BRITISH SUPPLEMENTS - *British supplements .net*

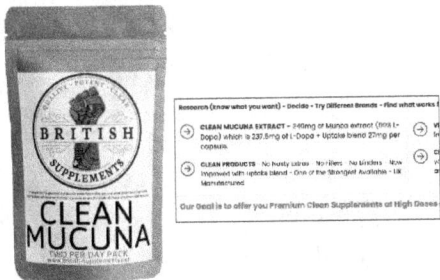

Capsule EXTRACT	99 %	1 caps = **237 mg** LD
seeds	240 mg	

This is the second most potent capsule. The extract from this laboratory, which advertises 99% levodopa, is available in capsules in two sizes (240 mg and 357 mg), and in powder packets (difficult to dose).

This page shows the capsule with 240 mg of extract, in which almost all of it is levodopa (237.6 mg), that is to say nearly as much as one Sinemet 25/250 (blue), or two and a half tablets of Sinemet Plus 25/100. It is useful for those who require high doses of levodopa.

BRITISH SUPPLEMENTS - British supplements . *net*

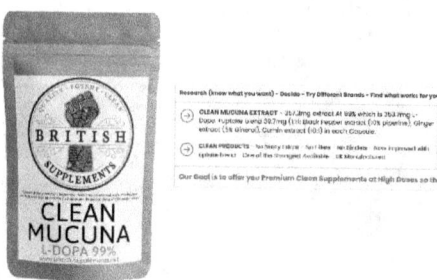

Capsule EXTRACT	99 %	1 caps = **353 mg** LD
seeds	357 mg	

Ultra-concentrated extract at 99%, no less than 353 mg of levodopa corresponding to 3 and a half tablets of Sinemet Plus, or the sum of one Sinemet Plus and one Sinemet 25/250. It adds 39.7 mg of extracts of black pepper, ginger and cumin, which is attributed to greater intestinal absorption of levodopa.

Patients say it is great, they feel very well, but they have to take the very high dose per capsule into consideration. Moreover, consisting of almost all levodopa, the capsules have lost most of the other components from the mucuna that are essential for its special effectiveness.

BRITISH SUPPLEMENTS - British supplements . *net*

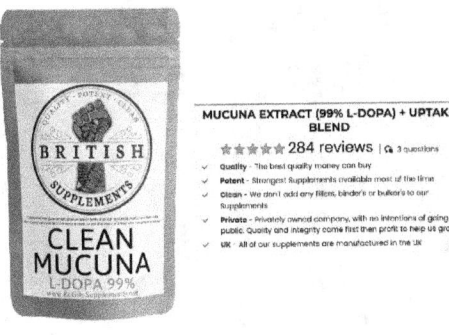

EXTRACT POWDER	99 %	1 tsp = **2970 mg?**
seeds	cup, 1/8	

The powder with 99% levodopa extract is very difficult to dose, they provide a small cup, 1/8 teaspoon (approximately 375 grams). If it contains that amount of levodopa, precision scales would be needed if we want to obtain 50 mg of levodopa, for example

Almost all of it is levodopa, namely 1 teaspoon (3 grams) would be 2970 mg of levodopa (like 30 Sinemet 25/100 tablets). It is surely dangerous, especially for those who have been taking pure powder (4%), of which a teaspoon contains only 120 mg.

CUREASE - *curease.com*

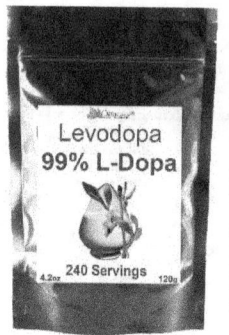
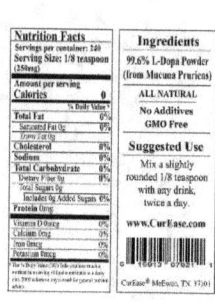

EXTRACT POWDER	99 %	1 tsp = **2000 mg?**
seeds	cup., 1/8 250 mg	

Powder with 99% seed extract. They provide a cup estimated to be 1/8 teaspoon (1/8 tsp) with 250 mg of levodopa.

They recommend servings of two cups (500 mg) twice a day: 1000 mg. According to their calculations, 1 teaspoon would have 8 times more than the cup, or 2000 mg of levodopa (like 20 Sinemet tablets without carbidopa).

NUTRIVITA powder - *nutrivitashop.com*

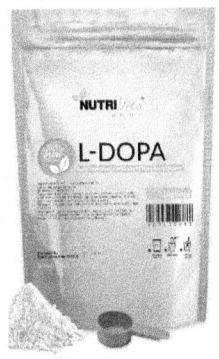
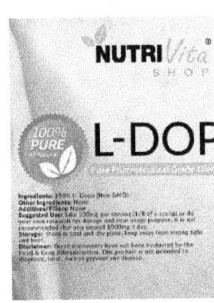

EXTRACT POWDER	100 %	1 tsp = **3000 mg?**
seeds	3 g	

Powder with 100% seed extract. The label suggests 500 mg per serving which is equivalent to 1/8 teaspoon or to "do your own research for dosage". If one-eighth of a cup is 500 mg of levodopa, for one cup you would have to multiply by 8 = 4000 mg of levodopa. Be careful with such high or confusing doses.

And if all what the powder contains is levodopa (are there any other ingredients left?), a teaspoon (3 grams) would be 3000 mg of levodopa. How would you dose for 50 or 100 mg?

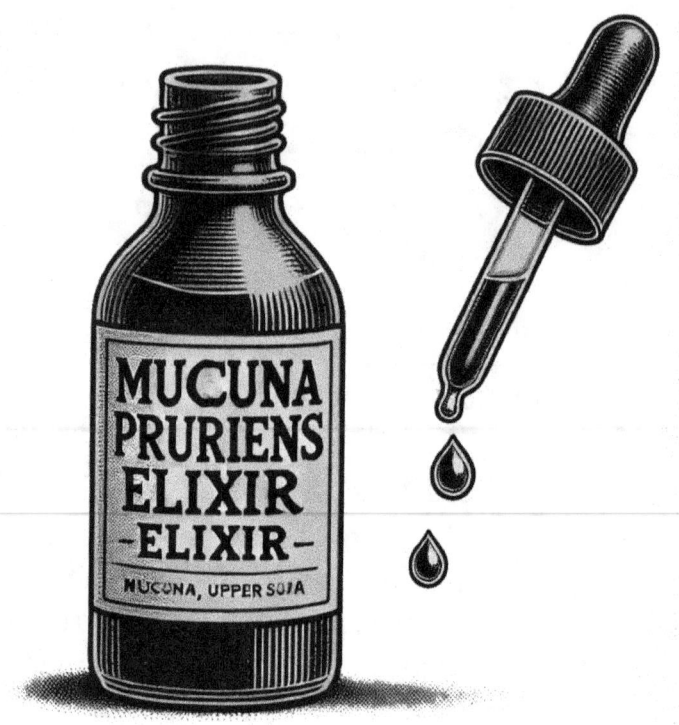

FIGURE 6: A little-known form of mucuna is its elixir, a liquid obtained from the seeds or the entire plant. The concentration of levodopa is usually low but offers a broader spectrum of its other bioactive compounds.

The seeds are dried, ground, macerated and filtered. The levodopa requirement can be completed with higher concentrations in capsules or powders.

8. Liquid extracts (elixirs)

An elixir is a sweet-tasting liquid used medicinally to cure diseases. When used as pharmaceutical preparation, it contains at least one active ingredient.

The manufacture of elixirs from natural products involves several steps that focus on the extraction of the active ingredients from plants, herbs or natural substances. These elixirs can have therapeutic, energetic or cosmetic purposes, and although there are various methods, most follow a basic process that includes the selection, extraction and preservation of the ingredients. Below, I will explain the typical process, applied to mucuna.

ELIXIR OF SEEDS OR THE WHOLE PLANT

The elixir can be derived from the seeds, which contain the highest amount of levodopa (L-dopa), or from the entire plant, including stems, leaves, and even roots, with the purpose of taking advantage of other therapeutic components. The levodopa content varies greatly depending on the part of the plant used:

Seeds contain between 3% and 7% levodopa, and its concentration varies depending on the plant variety, growing conditions, and stage of maturity at harvest. The whole plant spray contains little levodopa, between 0.5% and 1.5%, which makes it less effective.

However, it can offer a broader spectrum of bioactive compounds albeit with a much lower levodopa content.

PROCESS FOR MUCUNA ELIXIR

1. Plant selection

The first step in making a Mucuna Pruriens elixir is to choose high-quality plants, free of contaminants and correctly identified. It is crucial that the plants are mature and dry, since immaturity or humidity affect the stability and concentration of their active ingredients. Although in some cases other parts of the plant are used, we will focus here on the seeds.

2. Cleaning and drying

Seeds must be carefully cleaned to remove dirt or residue, either manually or using specialized equipment. They are then thoroughly air-dried in a clean environment or in a dehydrator at low temperature (maximum 40°C) to preserve their active compounds.

3. Grinding

Once dried, the seeds are ground into a fine powder, facilitating the release of active ingredients during maceration. This process must be carried out in a controlled environment to avoid the loss of volatile compounds.

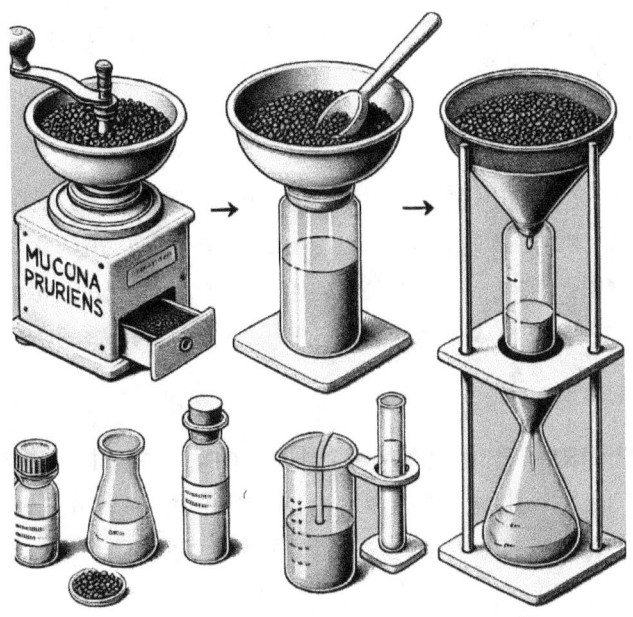

4. Maceration: extraction of active ingredients

Mucuna powder is macerated in high purity ethyl alcohol (ethanol), which is effective in extraction and has antimicrobial properties. The ethanol concentration varies between 70% and 96%, depending on the formulation. The standard ratio is 1:5 (one part powder to five parts solvent). The mixture is stored in dark glass bottles, shaking daily for 4 to 6 weeks to uniformly extract the active ingredients, such as levodopa.

5. Filtering and refining

After maceration, the mixture is filtered through a fine cloth or coffee filter to remove plant residues. A second filtering may be performed to ensure greater purity of the elixir.

6. Optional concentration

If a more concentrated product is sought, the filtered extract can be gently heated in a bain-marie to evaporate some of the alcohol, always controlling the temperature so as not to damage the levodopa.

7. Adjusting the formula

Ingredients, such as glycerin or honey, can be added to improve the flavour and stability of the elixir. Glycerin also acts as a natural preservative and reduces alcohol content.

8. Bottling and labeling

The elixir is bottled in dark glass bottles with droppers, previously sterilized, to protect it from light. It is important to label the product indicating ingredients, concentration, date of manufacture, expiration date and warnings for use.

9. Storage

The elixir should be stored in a cool, dark place to maintain its potency, with a shelf life of 1 to 3 years, depending on storage conditions.

10. Dosage; Standard doses are usually 10 to 20 sublingual drops, 1 or 2 times a day. However, the doctor may adjust the dosage according to the patient's needs, combining the elixir with more potent

mucuna extracts or with conventional drugs, if it contains little levodopa.

ELIXIR AND TINCTURE: DIFFERENCES

Tinctures are potent, unsweetened, high alcohol herbal extracts used in small doses.

Elixirs are milder, sweetened herbal solutions with lower alcohol content, designed for ease of consumption.

Both tinctures and elixirs are effective means of providing the therapeutic benefits of herbs, but the choice between them may depend on taste preferences, sensitivity to alcohol, and the specific needs of the individual.

COMMERCIAL ELIXIRS AND TINCTURES OF MUCUNA

They are difficult to find because they are rarely used. Some brands have stopped producing them due to low demand, but you can find some, like the ones described, Hawaii Pharm, Herbal Terra, Banyan, Absonutrix for the elixirs and Sun Potion for the tinctures.

HAWAI PHARM Elixir - *hawaiipharm.com*

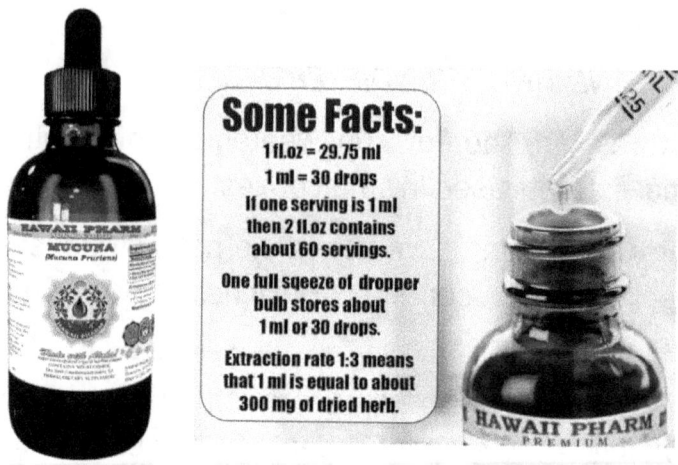

Elixir EXTRACT 1:3	4 %	1 ml = **12 mg** LD
seeds	300 mg	

The extraction method is interesting; they do not use alcohol but combine classical maceration with ultrasound. This way they obtain the equivalent of 300 mg of seeds, which at 4% gives us 12 mg of levodopa per milliliter.

HERBAL TERRA Elixir - *herbalterra.com*

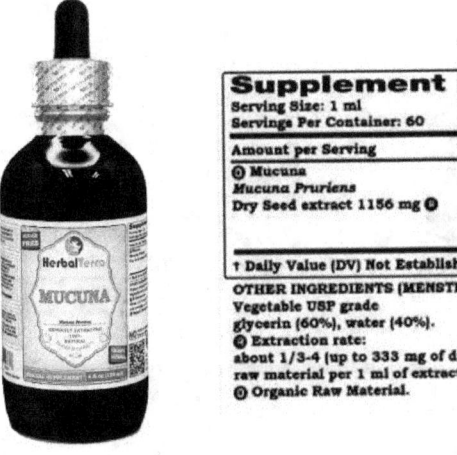

Elixir EXTRACT 1:3-4	4 %	1 ml = **13 mg** LD
seeds	333 mg	

This laboratory sells this elixir with glycerin and another with alcohol, with the same extraction power: 1156 mg of seeds in a 1: 3-4 ratio, and in 30 drops (1 ml) it would be equivalent to 333 mg. Estimating approximately 4% of levodopa, about 13 mg for 30 drops.

BANYAN Elixir – *banyanbotanicals.com*

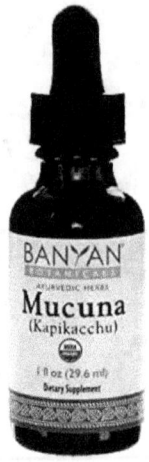
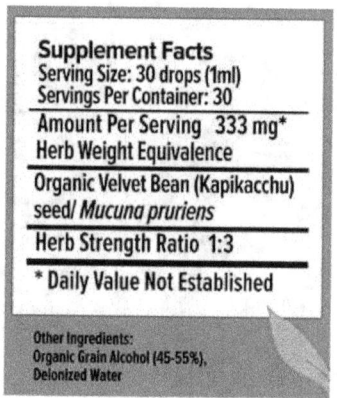

Elixir EXTRACT 1:3	4.5 %	1 ml = **15 mg** LD
seeds	333 mg	

Alcohol-based elixir that extracts in a 1:3 ratio up to the equivalent of 333 mg of seeds.

They report that the quality of their product ensures a 4.5% levodopa content, which would be 15 mg per milliliter (30 drops).

ABSONUTRIX Elixir - *amazon.com*

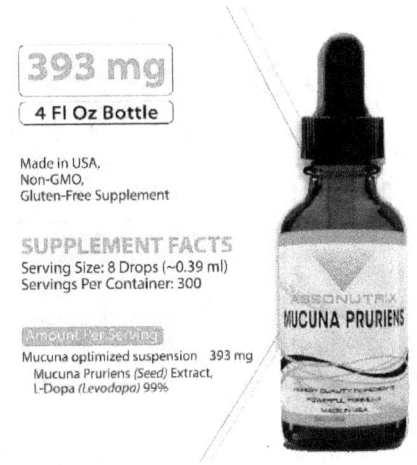

Elixir EXTRACT 1:?	4 %	1 ml = **39 mg** LD?
seeds	982 mg?	

They recommend a serving of 8 drops, which they calculate as 0.39 ml, so one milliliter would be 20 drops on your measuring cup. If that recommended dose is equivalent to 393 mg of seeds, at the usual 4%, it would contain 16 mg of levodopa.

That would be a super-concentrated elixir, compared to the others, because one milliliter (20 drops of your measuring cup) would contain 982 mg of the plant, which at 4% would be 39 mg of levodopa.

I wrote to them to clarify these points, but they replied evasively.

SUN POTION Tincture - *sunpotion.com*

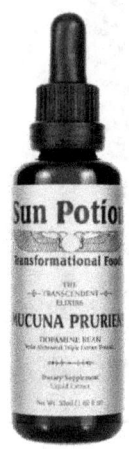
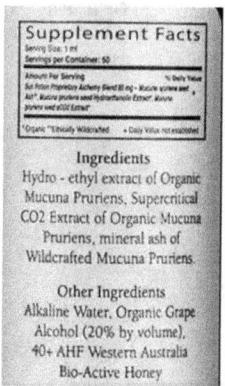

TINCTURE OF VARIOUS EXTRACTS

It is defined as very concentrated and expensive but no clear data on levodopa content is given.

This is the only mucuna tincture I have found. Tinctures are more concentrated than elixirs, with more alcohol, and without sweeteners or additives that change the taste. They are usually taken in very small doses. I have not found clear information about this one despite writing to the laboratory.

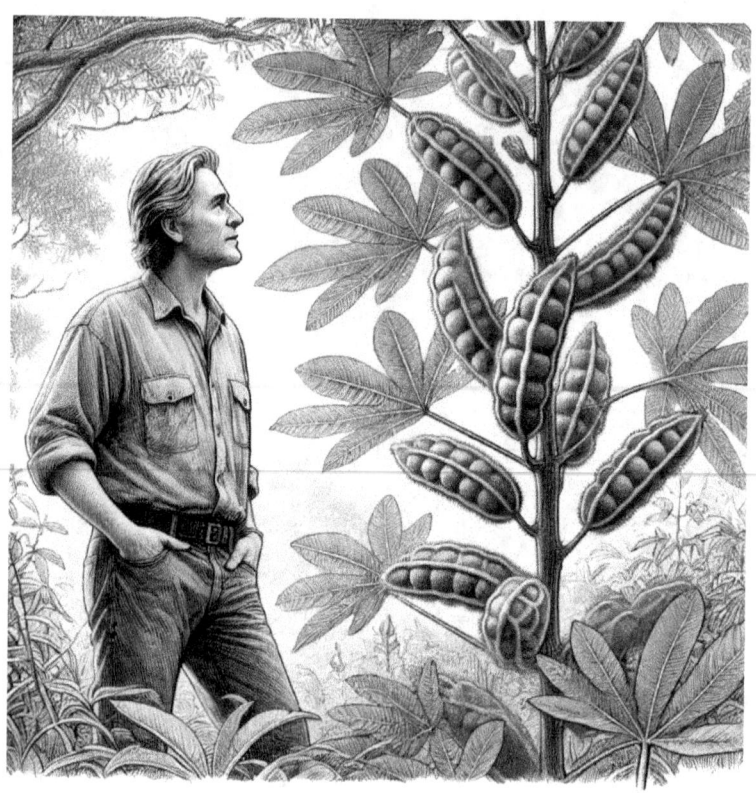

FIGURE 9. STARTING WITH MUCUNA.

Mucuna is a natural remedy, complementary in the treatment of Parkinson's. The first thing to do is to consult your doctor, and also to be well-informed about the issues that arise when you decide to start taking mucuna.

9. How to start with mucuna

Here I will give you some general information to discuss with your doctor, who will supervise your intake of mucuna and will be aware of the purpose for which it is used.

MUCUNA INDIVIDUAL PROFILE

The effectiveness of Mucuna pruriens varies from person to person, due to the complexity of its individual metabolism, which must be understood to optimize its use and minimize side effects.

This variability is similar to that observed with synthetic levodopa, but in the case of mucuna, the complexity is amplified due to its natural origin and the presence of multiple bioactive components.

WHAT INFLUENCES THE METABOLISM OF MUCUNA

1. Genetics: genes play a crucial role in how each person metabolizes mucuna. The enzymes dopamine decarboxylase and catechol-O-methyltransferase (COMT), which convert levodopa to dopamine, vary in efficiency depending on genetic variants, which affects the dosage needed.

2. Intestinal Microbiota: significantly influences the absorption of natural levodopa from mucuna.

Differences in bacterial composition can lead to very different responses between patients, even with the same dose.

3. Diet and Nutrition: protein-rich foods, for example, can compete with natural levodopa for the same transporters in the intestine and the blood-brain barrier, reducing its effectiveness. This is an aspect that is observed with both mucuna and synthetic levodopa. But legumes also have an influence, with consequences that also vary between individuals.

4. Psychological State and Stress: emotions modify the effectiveness of mucuna on symptoms. Stress and anxiety can alter intestinal absorption and the neurological response to dopamine, thus affecting the effectiveness of mucuna.

5. Evolutionary phase: as Parkinson's disease progresses, the metabolization profile of mucuna may change.

In the early stages, a lower dose of mucuna may be sufficient to control symptoms, while in more advanced stages, the patient may need adjustments in the dose or administration method to maintain efficacy.

This is what we also see with synthetic levodopa, where, over time, increasingly frequent adjustments have to be made.

VARIABLE RESPONSE ACCORDING TO MUCUNA

It is the same thing that we see with synthetic levodopa, whose response varies according to the person and the type of preparation: some improve more with Sinemet or Madopar, or with delayed forms, or additives such as entacapone or safinamide.

Mucuna, after all, is another way of administering levodopa, taking advantage of it with a different metabolization profile and efficacy. And it also varies according to the mucuna product used, which must be adapted to the patient and their stage of evolution.

VARIOUS PRESENTATIONS OF MUCUNA

Mucuna pruriens is available as pure seed powder, extracts of varying potency and powder, capsules or elixirs. It is also available in delayed-release forms, combining extracts of different concentrations, only seeds, from the whole plant, and even in gummies or tinctures for sublingual absorption.

Each of these forms may contain different concentrations of natural levodopa and other active compounds, which may affect their absorption and metabolism. Individual variability in response to these formulations may be significant, with some patients responding better to a specific form of mucuna while others prefer another.

THE OTHER COMPONENTS

Although mucuna is a natural source of levodopa, it is not simply a direct substitute for synthetic levodopa. It contains other components that may influence its absorption and metabolism, similarly to how carbidopa, benserazide, or entacapone affect synthetic levodopa.

CHOOSING THE MOST APPROPRIATE MUCUNA

The physician must decide on the most suitable mucuna preparation based on the individual patient's response. This means trying different types of preparations and dosages until the one that provides the greatest relief of symptoms with the fewest side effects is found. It is essential that patients listen to the signals their body is sending them and communicate with their physician for periodic adjustments.

PRACTICAL CASES

Starting mucuna in a patient who has not yet started antiparkinsonian drugs is relatively simple by following some basic instructions. I assume that the patient has no other relevant medical pathologies. I will describe some typical cases.

> **PATIENT 1:** *Between 40 and 80 years old. Recently diagnosed with Parkinson's disease. Mild symptoms. Has not yet taken any medication.*

Mucuna is an interesting option, but I recommend starting with it after the "shock" or grief phase that many patients experience when they find out they have Parkinson's disease.

It depends much on the way in which the patient has been told, whether it has been explained to him that there are many stages, different forms of evolution, and various treatment options. Sometimes the diagnosis sounds like a criminal sentence and the patient needs time to assimilate it. At that stage I prefer to wait, taking advantage of the opportunity to insist on exercise and other lifestyle recommendations.

Mucuna can be started later, always under the supervision of a doctor and having been well informed about the treatment and its possibilities.

PURE SEED POWDER (NO EXTRACTS)

First, the simplest mucuna should be used, the one that has been used for millennia. It has a low levodopa content, but it will suffice in these initial stages. There is no need to use extracts that always include artificial processing.

I recommend ZANDOPA first, at least the first bottle, because it is the mucuna that has been used in clinical trials, obtained from pulverized seeds with controlled quality standards.

There is currently a problem with the supply of Zandopa, due to customs controls or because there are seasons when the supply is interrupted. It can then be replaced by similar preparations (seed powder without complicated extracts) from other brands at a better price or more easily available.

Zandopa contains a 7.5 gram cup (about a teaspoon and a half) of seeds, which is equivalent to 250 milligrams of levodopa (an attempt was made to approximate the amount contained in a "blue" Sinemet 25/250).

I recommend starting slowly. Half a cup mid-morning (dissolved in water or juice), on an empty stomach. After 3-4 days, half a cup in the morning and another half in the afternoon.

This daily cup (half and a half) is 7.5 grams, approximately 250 mg of levodopa. But, as explained before, since it does not contain carbidopa, its effectiveness in improving symptoms is equivalent to a quarter, approximately 62.5 mg of levodopa (more or less, half of a Sinemet Plus 25/100). In other words, a great improvement cannot be expected and, probably, in this first phase, three half cups at least will be necessary.

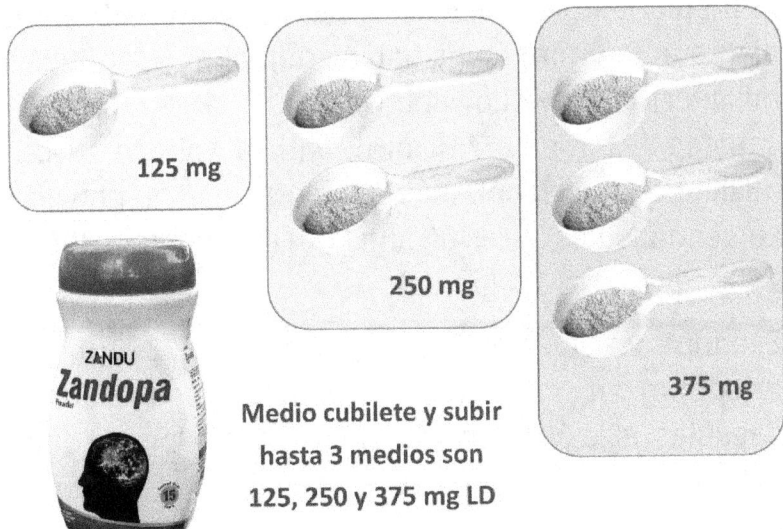

Medio cubilete y subir hasta 3 medios son 125, 250 y 375 mg LD

The disadvantage of seed powder is the taste, which some consider unpleasant, and the hassle of dissolving the powder. In these cases, the same product can be obtained in capsule form.

SEED POWDER CAPSULES

It is the same simple grinding of seeds, without chemical extracts or other manipulations, but to avoid the bad taste and the inconvenience of preparation, the powder has been introduced in capsules.

The problem is that the dosage is too small because the capsules cannot be too large. You would have to take several capsules per dose or the dose would be too low.

A medium-sized capsule (size 1, length 19 mm, diameter 6.6 mm) holds half a gram of powder (half a milliliter). A swallowable medium-large (size 0) capsule (21 mm x 7.3 mm), with a volume of 0.7 milliliters, may contain 680 milligrams of powder. Larger capsules (sizes 00 and 000) may contain 900 to 1400 mg (0.9 to 1.4 grams).

Zandopa vial (7.5 grams of powder with 250 mg of levodopa) in capsules, we would need 8 large capsules, size 00 (23 mm long) or 5 of the largest ones manufactured, size 000 (26 mm long).

If you find that mucuna powder works for you, but you find the taste unpleasant, and you have enough patience, you can buy empty capsules of the largest size that you can swallow to get the desired dosage. There are pharmacies that will do this for a reasonable price as well.

POWDER AND EXTRACTS IN CAPSULES

Because of these size and content difficulties, there are few brands with simple seed powder (there are many with extracts of different percentages).

Swanson capsules contain 400 mg of seed powder. Estimating a 4% percentage of levodopa, that's only 16 mg per capsule. It takes 15 to equal a shot glass, or 12 for one that holds a teaspoon or coffee spoon (5 grams).

Himalaya capsules are an interesting product because they combine, without extracts, mucuna seed and stem powder. The idea is to provide not only levodopa but also the other unknown substances that make the plant unique, by including it as a whole.

However, the amount of levodopa is greatly reduced because the stem (350 mg) has very little levodopa (0.25%) and together with the 250 mg of seeds (4%) there would only be 11-12 mg per capsule.

If you consider including the stem and only need a small amount of levodopa, you can take a large number of capsules (which would be expensive) or combine them with other capsules containing extracts with higher percentages of levodopa.

If 200-300 mg of natural levodopa are needed daily, it is preferable to use capsules with extracts, but with a low concentration (15-20%). Even so, 5-6 capsules will be necessary.

Zandopa's powder plan scheme would be:

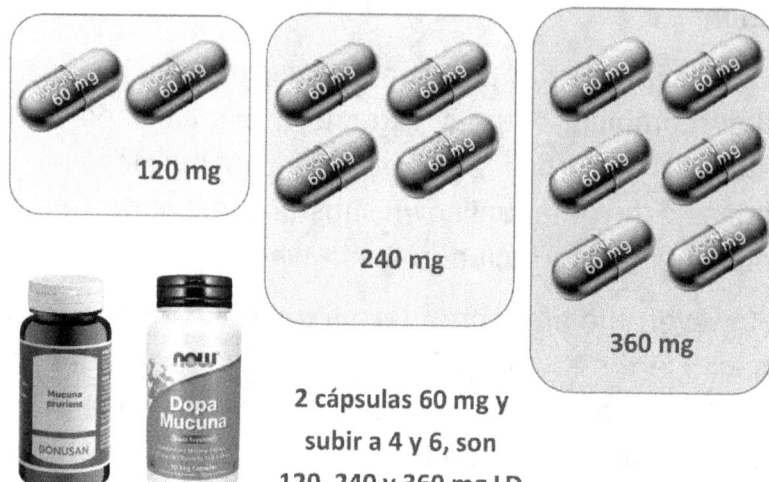

2 cápsulas 60 mg y subir a 4 y 6, son 120, 240 y 360 mg LD

Bonusan and Now are preparations with 60 mg and 15% extracts that fit this plan.

MONITOR THE RESPONSE

After starting the low dose, the patient's clinical response should be closely monitored, assessing both the improvement of motor symptoms and the emergence of possible side effects (such as nausea, gastrointestinal discomfort, or mild psychiatric symptoms).

Let us return to the example of Zandopa or other brands using simple seed powder:

If a daily cup (half in the morning and half in the afternoon = 250 mg of levodopa) is effective, this could be continued for weeks or months, and then increased.

DOSE ADJUSTMENTS IN PERIODIC CONSULTATIONS

It is advisable to schedule frequent follow-up visits to assess progress and adjust the dosage as necessary. If the patient tolerates the initial dose well and improvement is noted, a gradual increase in the dose in small increments (e.g., increasing by 1-2 grams each week) may be considered up to the maximum, which will be established by the physician after observing the improvement of symptoms and possible side effects.

In these early stages of the disease, combination with other antiparkinsonian drugs should be avoided. Since the patient has not yet started any treatment with synthetic levodopa, it is preferable to first try mucuna pruriens as monotherapy before considering any combination.

MONOTHERAPY WITH MUCUNA

Using mucuna pruriens as monotherapy in the early stages of Parkinson's may not only delay the need for synthetic levodopa, but also reduce the occurrence of common side effects associated with conventional treatments. Research suggests that this strategy may offer a better long-term quality of life for patients.

> **PATIENT 2.** *Between 40 and 80 years old, with moderate symptoms. She has not yet taken any medication. She is doing well with Mucuna, but it is insufficient.*

This patient with moderate symptoms insists on not taking any drugs. She started with a low dose of mucuna pruriens powder (Zandopa), with 7.5 grams daily divided into two doses. She then increased the dose to three half-cups (about 11 grams per day of seeds, 375 mg of levodopa). Although she has shown a clear improvement, this is still insufficient.

This is usual because much larger amounts have been used in a single dose in clinical trials in patients; 30 grams of powder (1000 mg of levodopa) improved symptoms more than one Sinemet 25/250 tablet, with fewer adverse effects (Katzenschlager 2004, Cilia 2017).

I recommend much lower doses in the early stages of the disease.

It may be sufficient to gradually increase to 3 scoops of Zandopa or equivalent, spread throughout the day: 22.5 grams (750 mg of levodopa) in one day, which is less than the 30 grams given in a single dose in the trials.

INCREASED DOSE OF MUCUNA

Since the patient has responded well to the initial dose, you may consider gradually increasing the dose to 10-15 grams daily divided into two doses (morning and evening). This would involve 1 full scoop of Zandopa in the morning and another in the evening, corresponding to 15 grams daily. This adjustment should be done under the supervision of the physician, paying particular attention to the clinical response and possible side effects.

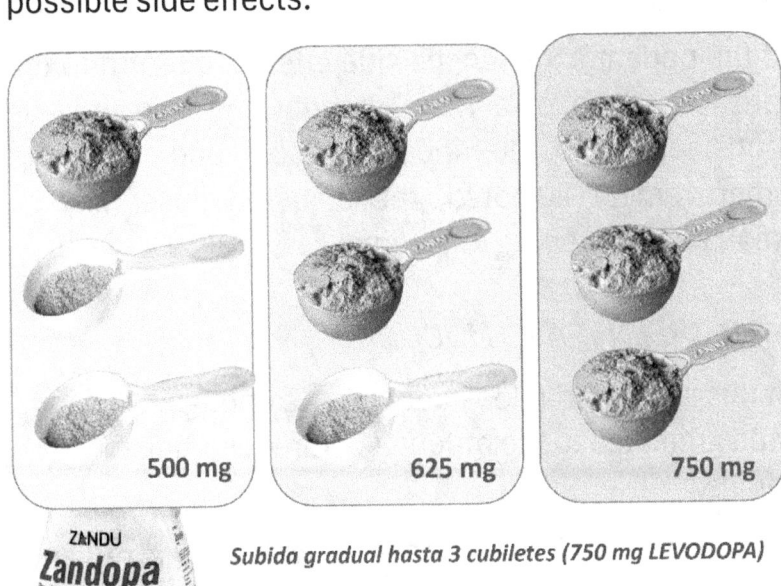

Subida gradual hasta 3 cubiletes (750 mg LEVODOPA)

If the symptoms have barely improved, the dose could be gradually increased to two or even three cups a day. With three cups a day of Zandopa, you are taking 22.5 grams of seeds (750 mg of levodopa) but its benefit on the symptoms is less than a quarter of the amount of synthetic levodopa (187.5 mg), which would be less than one Sinemet 25/250 (three quarters of a tablet).

CONTROL RESPONSE AND TOLERANCE

As always, after dose adjustment, it is crucial that the patient is closely observed for any changes in motor and non-motor symptoms, as well as the emergence of adverse effects such as nausea, dyskinesias or mild psychiatric symptoms.

If the patient experiences side effects, a return to the previous dose or a more gradual increase may be considered. If tolerance is good and symptom improvement is noted, the adjusted dose may be maintained over the long term.

ADD GREEN TEA TO MUCUNA

If this patient still does not improve enough, we can add green tea to the mucuna before resorting to drugs.

Green tea is rich in polyphenols with recognized antioxidant and neuroprotective properties and some, such as EGCG (epigallocatechin gallate), have been shown to have inhibitory properties on dopa decarboxylase, an action similar to that of carbidopa although much weaker.

This may enhance the effects of mucuna pruriens by allowing more levodopa to cross the blood-brain barrier, where it is converted into dopamine.

Therefore, tea infusions, once or twice a day, preferably together with mucuna doses, may improve symptoms to some extent.

Another option is to use green tea extract in capsule or concentrate form, assuring that the product contains sufficient EGCG content, but they should not be used without medical supervision because some extracts are too concentrated and, although they improve the effectiveness of levodopa, they cause interactions with other medications and can aggravate underlying medical pathologies.

> **PATIENT 3.** *Symptoms are already significant and affect daily life. They improve with mucuna, but need a lot of dosage, with concentrated extracts and combined with green tea but still insufficient.*

Mucuna is not an alternative treatment but a complementary one. Drugs should be started late and at the lowest possible dose, especially at the beginning, but sooner or later they will have to be taken since you cannot be an extremist about anything, not even about natural therapies.

This patient was determined not to stop by the pharmacy. He exercised, changed his lifestyle, and thanks to his praiseworthy efforts has saved 2-3 years of drugs. Unfortunately, now mucuna is not enough for him, as well as the carbidopa effect of green tea, despite taking it in strong extracts. He tried to get carbidopa alone (Lodosyn), which is sold in 25-mg tablets, but it was not possible since it is only sold in the USA or Canada and unfortunately not in Europe. Zandopa being too weak, he is now trying to solve the problem by taking highly concentrated extracts of mucuna (70 to 99% levodopa).

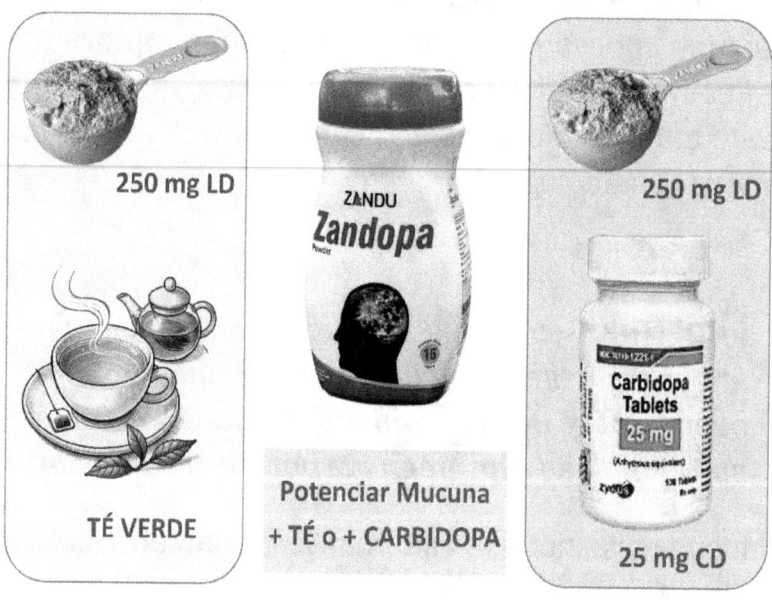

In fact, the mucuna from Zandopa was shown here to be insufficient and there was not much improvement when adding green tea extracts (it was previously confirmed that there had been no polypathologies or drugs with which they suspected interactions).

MUCUNA WITH A LITTLE SINEMET

If after gradual titration mucuna pruriens is still insufficient, the addition of a small dose of synthetic levodopa (such as levodopa/carbidopa) may be considered in the future. This would only be necessary if symptoms are not adequately controlled with mucuna alone.

The combination of mucuna pruriens with synthetic levodopa has been investigated in several studies and has been found to be particularly useful in patients who do not respond completely to mucuna alone. However, this combination should be handled with care to avoid the occurrence of serious side effects, such as dyskinesias, which are more common with prolonged use of levodopa.

It is time to combine mucuna with small amounts of Sinemet or Madopar to take advantage of the carbidopa and benserazide they contain respectively. Even in small amounts, they will enhance both the synthetic levodopa and the natural levodopa in mucuna.

This combination will allow you to save on mucuna (which was already a high expense due to the high doses) and, above all, it will reduce the already very high amount of natural levodopa you were taking (or not so much, because ultra-concentrated extracts have powerful chemical methods that distort the original qualities of the plant, precisely those that give its superior benefits).

QUARTER OF MADOPAR OR HALF SINEMET PLUS?

Carbidopa and benserazide are very similar, but they are not the same. Some patients do better with one or even a combination of them.

¼ Madopar 50/200 = ½ Sinemet 25/100

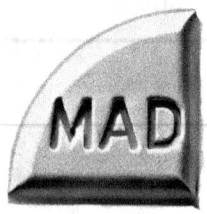

LEVODOPA
50 mg

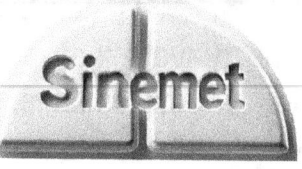

BENSERAZIDA 12,5 mg   CARBIDOPA 12,5 mg

Algo más rápida   Algo más duradera

I usually start with benserazide, which seems to have a faster effect although it is less long-lasting. In addition, patients are more convinced by a quarter of a Madopar tablet than by half a Sinemet Plus, which contains the same amount of synthetic levodopa (50 mg).

In order to obtain 12.5 mg of benserazide or carbidopa, patients will have to "endure" 50 mg of synthetic levodopa. However, it is not that much, and the mixture is very beneficial.

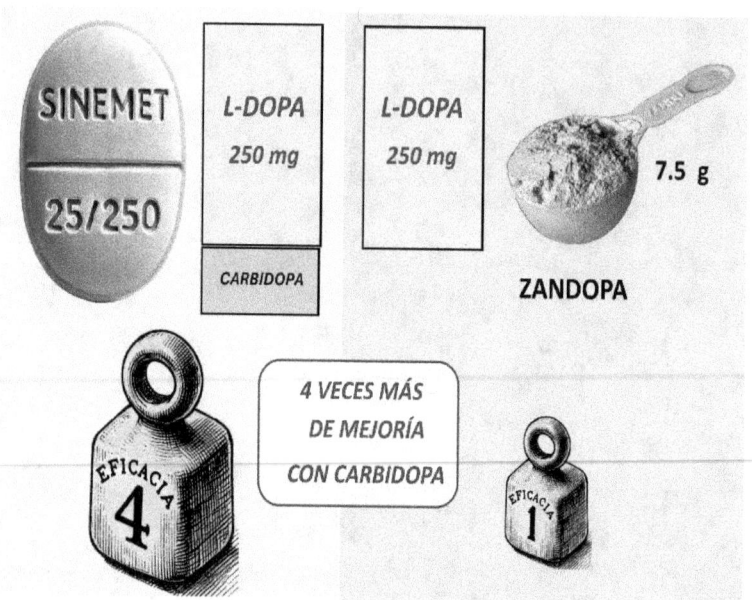

FIGURE 9. It is difficult to adjust the dose of mucuna. A Sinemet 25/250 contains 250 mg of synthetic levodopa, like the 250 mg of natural levodopa in a Zandopa cup (7.5 grams of seed powder). But since mucuna does not contain carbidopa, its effect on symptoms is a quarter of that.

1,000 mg of natural levodopa (30 grams of seed powder) is needed for the effect of one Sinemet 25/250 tablet... unless carbidopa is added to the mucuna. Be careful when combining them, because the carbidopa in the tablet potentiates the mucuna: consult your doctor!

10. Combining mucuna and drugs

Mucuna pruriens is not an alternative treatment but a complementary treatment for Parkinson's disease. It should always be used under medical supervision, especially if you plan to reduce some of your antiparkinsonian medications.

Only a portion of synthetic levodopa can be replaced by the natural levodopa present in mucuna, and a dose of carbidopa or benserazide (which potentiate the effect of levodopa) must be maintained. Dopamine agonists and other antiparkinsonian drugs may still be necessary, at least in part; if they are decreased, the drug must compensate for this by increasing the dose of levodopa, whether synthetic or natural.

In advanced stages of the disease, these changes may be more complicated because the drugs act on different areas of the brain. Levodopa acts on the *substantia nigra*, which is necessary for converting it into dopamine, but which deteriorates over time. Dopamine agonists act in the *striatum*, offering an alternative route to the nigrostriatal pathway and functioning as a shortcut that is sometimes essential.

In the initial stages, when symptoms are mild and treatment is based on synthetic levodopa (such as Sinemet, Madopar or Stalevo), it is possible to partially replace this with natural levodopa from mucuna.

However, it is advisable to maintain a small dose of synthetic levodopa so that mucuna can benefit from the carbidopa or benserazide in the drug.

PREVIOUS STEPS

Before introducing mucuna there are some steps to take:

- Review general medication to prevent interactions or complications, eliminating those that are not necessary.

- Calculate the amount of carbidopa or benserazide you were taking and the amount you will continue taking to enhance mucuna.

- Assess whether there are other antiparkinsonian drugs that can be reduced and how their absence will be compensated.

- Plan the schedule for adjustments. A period of time should be chosen when the patient and his/her doctor are available, without other occupations that prevent frequent consultations for successive adjustments.

CONSIDER THE INDIVIDUAL RESPONSE

Response to mucuna varies from patient to patient. Close monitoring during the first few days of use is crucial. This allows any adverse effects or lack of efficacy to be detected and managed in a timely manner.

SMALL DOSES AND PERIODIC ADJUSTMENTS

Previous symptoms will be assessed, how they change when introducing mucuna, especially the first days or weeks, and any relevant changes, positive or negative, will be recorded.

Initially, mucuna doses will be low, gradually increasing based on patient tolerance and clinical response. Based on the observed response, adjust the mucuna dose to optimize symptom control without causing adverse effects. This may involve gradual increases or decreases.

Blood pressure and heart function will be reviewed, as well as the variations that may occur with other pathologies and medications.

DOPAMINERGIC AGONISTS

Special care must be taken when changing the dosage. In elderly patients, dopamine agonists can cause significant side effects, such as sleep disorders or cognitive impairment.

However, reducing them can cause decompensations that the doctor should have anticipated.

CONTINUOUS MONITORING

A gradual plan will have been designed for any pharmacological change, ensuring that the motor symptoms of Parkinson's continue to be effectively controlled.

The patient's response will be monitored closely and periodically, with adjustments as necessary to maintain an optimal balance between efficacy and tolerability.

PART OF LEVODOPA MAY BE FLEXIBLE

The physician will stop some of the treatment at fixed times (essential slow-acting or single-dopa forms) but some of the levodopa may be left to the patient's discretion within a narrow window. This "levodopa *ad libitum* " approach allows them to partially adjust the dose and schedule for individual symptom management.

PRACTICAL CASES

The doctor may recommend a partial and gradual replacement of synthetic levodopa with natural levodopa from mucuna pruriens, following the general information and practical examples presented below.

For substitutions, mucuna capsules with low concentration extracts of levodopa (15-20%) are recommended. These products maintain most of the plant components and have a smaller volume. Some options are Dopabean (50 mg of levodopa per capsule), Dopamucuna and Bonusan (60 mg of levodopa per capsule).

We will use Dopabean as a reference, as its 50mg levodopa content makes calculations easier. Other products with different levodopa concentrations, such as Pure Encapsulation (10mg), Advance Physician (30 mg) or DoubleWood (100 mg) may also be used with dosages adjusted as needed.

CASE 1: REDUCE SINEMET PLUS 25/100

The person uses Sinemet Plus 25/100 tablets daily and wants to change part of them to mucuna.

Knowing that a Sinemet Plus 25/100 tablet contains 25 mg carbidopa and 100 mg levodopa, I suggest he take Sinemet Plus tablets with two Dopabean capsules (50 mg levodopa per capsule). However, since mucuna does not contain carbidopa, the clinical effect would be weaker, only partly compensated by the carbidopa in the previous doses.

What I recommend is a partial substitution, namely changing the Sinemet Plus 25/100 tablet (25 mg carbidopa, 100 mg levodopa) for half a Sinemet 25/100 tablet (12.5 mg carbidopa and 50 mg levodopa) and a Dopabean capsule (50 mg natural levodopa).*

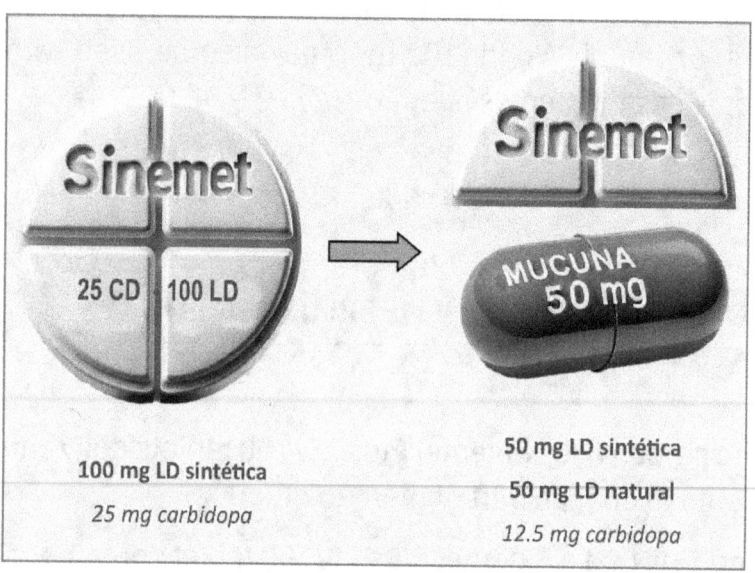

100 mg LD sintética
25 mg carbidopa

50 mg LD sintética
50 mg LD natural
12.5 mg carbidopa

Thus, the 100 mg synthetic levodopa has been changed to 50 mg synthetic and 50 mg natural, maintaining 12.5 mg of carbidopa, which will be sufficient to enhance the combination of the two.

---

*There is no need to be so exact, instead of the 50 mg capsules you can use 60 mg levodopa capsules, such as those from Bonusan and Now Foods.

CASE 2: REDUCE MADOPAR 50/200

A patient takes three tablets of Madopar 50/200 daily and wishes to introduce Mucuna pruriens into his treatment.

The procedure will be the same as described with Sinemet 25/100, assuming that it is equivalent to half a Madopar 50/200 if we consider carbidopa and benserazide to be alike. To facilitate the calculation, I have readapted it.

Madopar 50/200 tablet contains 50 mg benserazide and 200 mg levodopa. Your doctor may decide to change one of these doses. One Madopar 50/200 tablet could be replaced by four Dopabean capsules (each containing 333 mg *mucuna pruriens* with 15% levodopa, i.e. 50 mg levodopa per capsule) but, since *mucuna pruriens* does not contain benserazide, the clinical effect will be weaker, poorly compensated by the action of benserazide from the previous Madopar dose.

What I recommend is a partial substitution, namely changing the Madopar 50/200 tablet (50 mg carbidopa, 200 mg levodopa) for half a Madopar 50/200 tablet (50 benserazide and 100 mg levodopa) and two Dopabean capsules (100 mg natural levodopa).

Thus, the 200 mg of synthetic levodopa have been replaced by 100 mg synthetic and 100 mg natural levodopa, while maintaining 50 mg of benserazide, which will be sufficient to enhance the combination of the two.

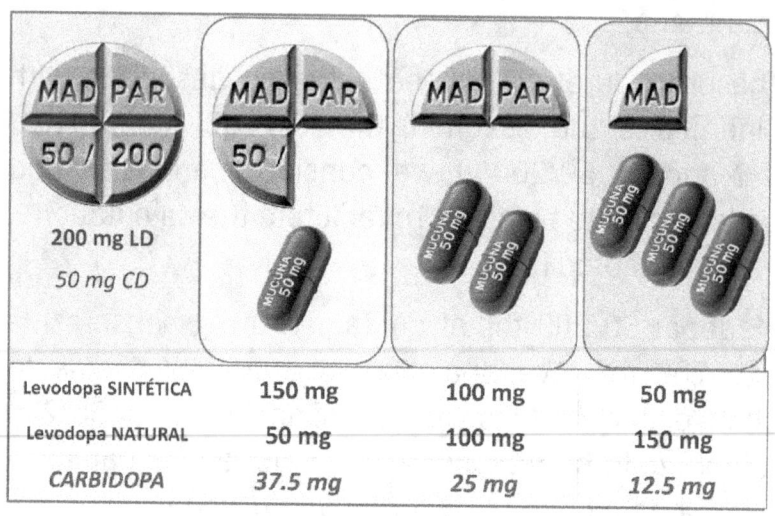

Levodopa SINTÉTICA	150 mg	100 mg	50 mg
Levodopa NATURAL	50 mg	100 mg	150 mg
CARBIDOPA	37.5 mg	25 mg	12.5 mg

I recommend that the doctor, following these calculations, propose the change in two stages: first reduce the Madopar tablet to ¾ of a tablet, adding a Dopabean (150 mg synthetic levodopa and 50 mg natural), and the 37.5 mg benserazide would be sufficient for both. In a second step, the change would be made to half a Madopar tablet.

Afterwards and only if the response is good, the doctor might propose to gradually increase the proportion of mucuna pruriens in the treatment but keep some benserazide. I recommend keeping a quarter of a Madopar tablet (12.5 mg benserazide and 50 mg levodopa in each dose) to be compensated with 150 mg of natural levodopa from the three Dopabean capsules.

CASE 3: REDUCE SINEMET 25/250

A patient takes Sinemet 25/250 tablets daily and is seeking to introduce mucuna. The carbidopa/levodopa ratio being 1:10, if we follow the above guidelines, we will be left with a quarter of Sinemet 25/250. Therefore, we would have only 6.25 mg carbidopa to enhance 62.5 mg of synthetic levodopa and 187.5 mg of natural levodopa would be missing as compensation (approximately 4 Dopabean capsules).

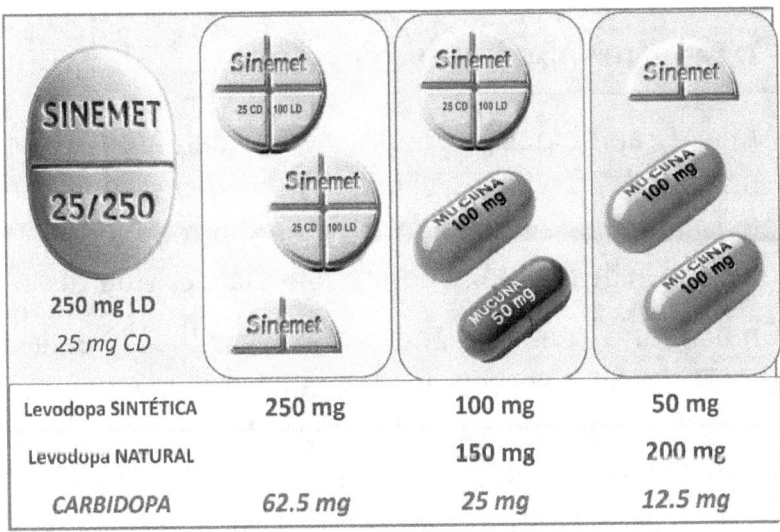

Levodopa SINTÉTICA	250 mg	100 mg	50 mg
Levodopa NATURAL		150 mg	200 mg
CARBIDOPA	62.5 mg	25 mg	12.5 mg

This problem is relatively easy to solve. Since we need more carbidopa, the doctor will recommend a first step as simple as changing one Sinemet 25/250 tablet for its equivalent in Sinemet 25/100, namely two and a half tablets. We thus maintain the 250 mg of levodopa but enriched with 62.5mg carbidopa.

After this substitution, you can gradually reduce the two and a half tablets of Sinemet 25/100 using the above guidelines.

An intermediate step can be saved by replacing the Sinemet 25/250 tablet with only half (12.5 mg carbidopa, 125 mg levodopa), plus a Sinemet 25/100 tablet totaling 37.5 mg carbidopa and 225 mg levodopa, eventually adding a mucuna containing 25-30 mg of natural levodopa (Advance Physician, for example).

CASE 4: PATIENTS TAKING STALEVO

Stalevo combines levodopa with carbidopa and entacapone, which significantly increases the bioavailability of levodopa. The introduction of mucuna in this context requires special consideration.

Entacapone inhibiting another enzyme that is called COMT, it will also potentiate the natural levodopa in mucuna. Together with carbidopa, the result is less predictable but is usually upward.

Stalevo 100 is equivalent to Sinemet Plus 25/100 plus 200 mg entacapone, giving a total of 100 mg levodopa together with 25 mg carbidopa and 200 mg entacapone.

The simplest option is to replace one Stalevo 100 tablet with one Stalevo 50 (50 mg levodopa, 12.5 mg carbidopa and 200 mg entacapone) together with one Dopabean capsule (50 mg levodopa).

CASE 5: RELUCTANT TO TAKE CARBIDOPA

Some patients are so serious about avoiding any drug that they abuse natural ones. This would be the case of the staunch enemy of carbidopa who clings to the well-known 1:4 ratio of the clinical effect between synthetic levodopa (with carbidopa) and natural levodopa from mucuna (without carbidopa). This relationship is true, but only in the absence of any carbidopa, and only in relation to the expected improvement of symptoms.

In their interpretation, they believe that if they substitute, for example, a Sinemet 25/250 mg for 1000 mg of mucuna levodopa, they only take 250 mg of levodopa. No, since it is evident that with four cups of pure seed powder (like Zandopa), 1000 mg of natural levodopa will be reaching their body. It is clearly less toxic and its side effects are mild, these two elements being supported by three millennia of traditional use and recent clinical trials (in which much higher doses are given).

But it is 1000 mg, they cannot fool themselves, and worse when those 1000 mg do not come from simple ground seeds but from extracts in high percentages, up to 99% of levodopa. In these ultra-concentrates there is hardly any plant left, only levodopa, almost like the synthetic one. And even worse if they combine them on their own (always consult a doctor) with carbidopa in more or less quantity, and when they mix with other antiparkinsonian drugs.

I recommend maintaining the priority of natural levodopa but boosting it with a very low dose of carbidopa to lower mucuna. That minimum carbidopa (let's say 12.5 mg of Sinemet 25/100) would not be enough to quadruple the potency of mucuna, but perhaps double it or something similar, depending on the individual metabolism.

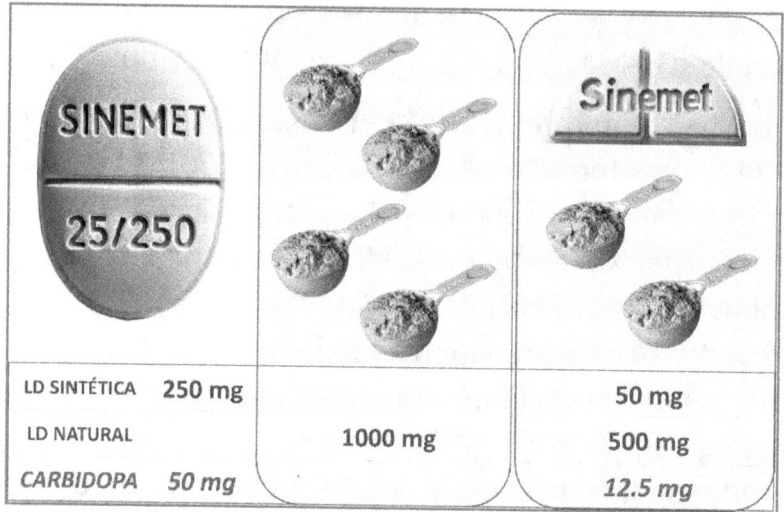

LD SINTÉTICA 250 mg		50 mg
LD NATURAL	1000 mg	500 mg
CARBIDOPA 50 mg		12.5 mg

In the indicated case, I would test how the patient reacts to replacing the 1000 mg of seed powder that he had been taking with half (500 mg) which, together with 12.5 mg of carbidopa and 50 mg of half a Sinemet 25/100 tablet, could improve his condition sufficiently with a balanced proportion, limiting the side effects.

CASE 6: PATIENTS WITH DYSKINESIAS

For motor fluctuations, Olanow proposed short, frequent doses of a levodopa solution. This stabilizes plasma levels, improves clinical response, and reduces *off* and freezing.

Mucuna spoils quickly in water (it turns black), so it must be taken quickly after diluting it, and it would be cumbersome.

A simpler option is to use capsule preparations with a low concentration of levodopa, for example, the aforementioned Advance Physician (30 mg levodopa per capsule) or even capsules without extract, which only contain the simple seed powder (Swanson, about 16 mg levodopa) or a mixture of powdered seeds and stem (Himalaya, about 11 mg), or, if necessary, 50 mg (Dopabean, Bonusan).

This would be added to a fixed medication combining conventional levodopa: delayed forms (Sinemet CR 25/100) in a fixed dose morning and night (to maintain a minimum of levodopa in the blood at any time, combined with 5 mucuna capsules spaced apart (15 to 50 mg depending on the case) and, for example, three doses of Sinemet 25/100 of half or one tablet (depending on the case), but administered in a flexible way: advance the dose if it is blocked, delay it a little if dyskinesias.

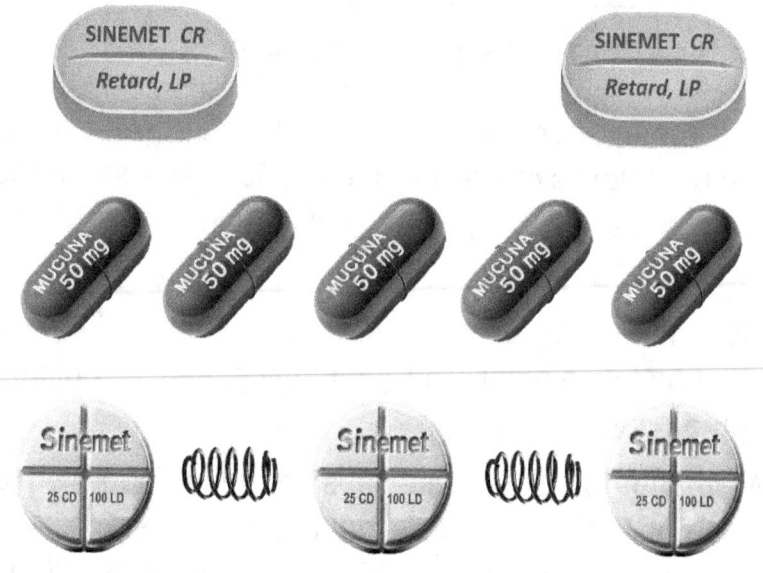

In some cases or stages, it is combined with agonists or other antiparkinsonian drugs that may be necessary at this stage.

The doctor will calculate the number and frequency of doses after listening to the patient and monitor the variations every few days.

CASE 7: VERY ADVANCED PATIENTS

In advanced patients with dyskinesias and other complications, some attempt to decrease the carbidopa ratio by increasing the synthetic levodopa. Others have tried to switch quickly from conventional carbidopa preparations to mucuna. They came with very high doses of synthetic levodopa which was replaced by four times as much mucuna levodopa.

Clinical efficacy was similar, but half of the patients did not tolerate such a rapid change (CILIA 2018). This should be done gradually, or by combining carbidopa with mucuna. In cases where high doses of medication are needed, seed powder is not sufficient.

It should be taken in large quantities and nausea and flatulence cause its withdrawal. Various conventional drugs must be maintained and, if it is decided to combine it with mucuna, ultra-concentrated preparations would be useful here, preferably in capsules rather than in powder form, which is more difficult to dose, with the risk of overdose. In these cases, the direction of the doctor we have indicated throughout this book is especially important. The information in this book is the one that the doctor must evaluate and decide on the options.

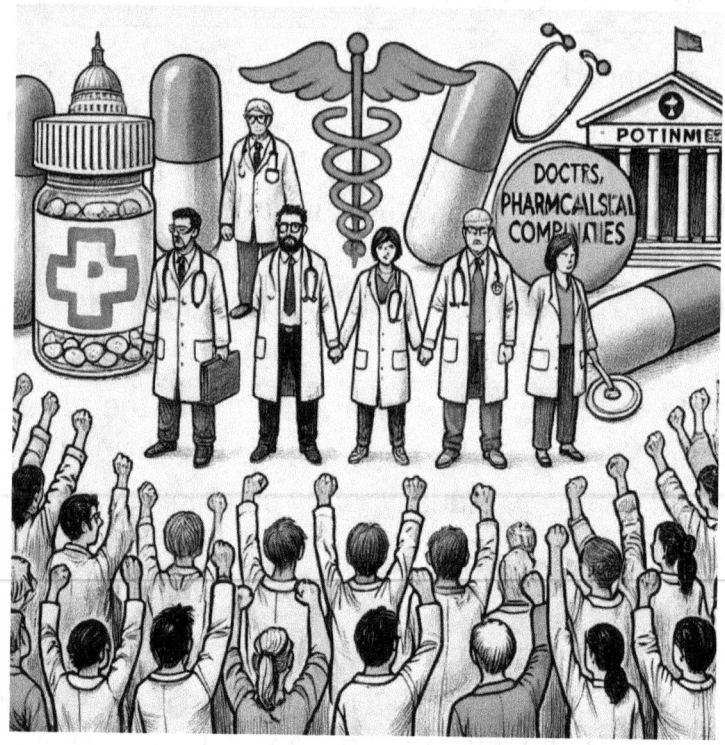

FIGURE 11. Patient forums are used to voice their demands. The state does not investigate enough, and many doctors barely listen to them, especially when they ask about natural remedies, which they use secretly.

They discuss this among themselves, learning from their experiences, but without medical supervision there is a risk of making mistakes. These concerns were brought to my attention by Marianne van der Meer (Mucuna Pruriens Parkinson forum) and Jérôme Simonin (renowned translator of books on Parkinson's).

11. Patients lose their patience (Patient forum)

(Collaborators: Marianne van der Meer and Jérôme Simonin)

Patient forums and associations do much more than just supporting groups. In the case of people with Parkinson's disease, they have become real spaces of resistance. People do not only share their experiences, but also raise their voices against a system that, they feel, has left them aside.

A rebellion is beginning. We are not just talking about consolation here; we are faced with a platform where they debate, question and, yes, even organize to demand what they consider fair. And at the center of many of these conversations is Mucuna pruriens, a plant that promises much and generates almost as many doubts as hopes.

WIDESPREAD DISCONTENT

Will someone please listen? The discomfort of Parkinson's patients is obvious, and it is not difficult to understand why. Their complaints revolve around three main points that emerge again and again in the discussions of these forums:

1. Lack of research: Where are the funds for Parkinson's research? Patients are tired of always hearing the same thing: that progress is limited, that there are not enough resources, that a cure is still far away. Meanwhile, life goes on, and those affected feel that time is running out.

2. Doctors are out of touch: A common criticism is that doctors seem to have a pre-established playbook: they come in, prescribe the same drugs and that's it. Listening to patients, tailoring treatments to their needs or even considering their concerns seems to be, in many cases, a rare exception. It's no wonder so many patients turn to forums in search of something more.

3. Disdain for natural treatments: many patients have found relief in natural medicine, but when they mention it to their doctors, the response is a resounding "that doesn't work." Mucuna pruriens, which contains levodopa, is a clear example.

Although some patients claim that it helps with their symptoms, most doctors ignore it or simply dismiss it. And sometimes they may be disregarding what they do not know because it is difficult to calculate the dosages, and they haven't had time to study them.

MUCUNA: SALVATION OR FALSE HOPE?

Among the natural remedies most often mentioned on forums is Mucuna pruriens. This plant, rich in levodopa (yes, the same compound found in many traditional Parkinson's medications), has raised expectations among patients. However, its use comes with its own set of problems:

1. Medical ignorance: although it contains levodopa, mucuna is not part of "official" treatments. Doctors do not know how to dose it or what long-term effects it may have. For many patients, this is a huge obstacle and they feel like they are exploring uncharted territory alone.

2. What is really in the products? A very serious problem is the quality of mucuna products that are marketed. Some patients have noticed that the levels of levodopa advertised do not always match the real ones, generating distrust. The demand is clear: mandatory certificates of analysis so that patients know what they are taking.

3. Lack of information: both doctors and patients are, in many cases, sailing blindly. There is not enough reliable information on how to use mucuna safely and effectively. Forums, in this sense, are a refuge where patients exchange experiences, but the lack of solid studies leaves many questions unanswered.

WHY HIDE WHAT WORKS?

It is worrying that many patients do not dare to tell their doctors that they are using natural products. The reason? They fear being judged or, worse, scolded.

This reflects a serious problem in the doctor-patient relationship: the lack of mutual trust. If patients cannot speak openly about what they are trying or how they feel, it is very difficult to move towards a personalized and effective treatment.

AN UNDERVALUED SOURCE OF KNOWLEDGE

Beyond emotional relief, patient forums and associations emerge as an invaluable source of data to understand what is working and what is not. Why not conduct surveys?

By systematically collecting patients' experiences, crucial data could be obtained on the benefits and risks of alternative treatments such as mucuna. This would help to reduce the knowledge gap between doctors and their patients and allow Parkinson's patients to be addressed in a more comprehensive way.

CALL TO ACTION

It is time for the health system to start paying attention to what these patients are saying. It is not just about prescribing pills or following the same old treatments. Parkinson's patients deserve to be heard, and their experiences with treatments such as mucuna must be taken seriously. Otherwise, they will continue to turn to forums to find the answers that, for now, they do not obtain in consultations.

CONCLUSIONS

Parkinson's patient forums are no longer just spaces for complaints. They are authentic platforms for empowerment where those affected share experiences, fight against the system and seek alternative solutions. To improve the quality of life of these patients, it is essential that doctors and researchers take note and value what is happening in these spaces. Because, in the end, if we do not listen to those who live with the disease every day, who are we really helping?

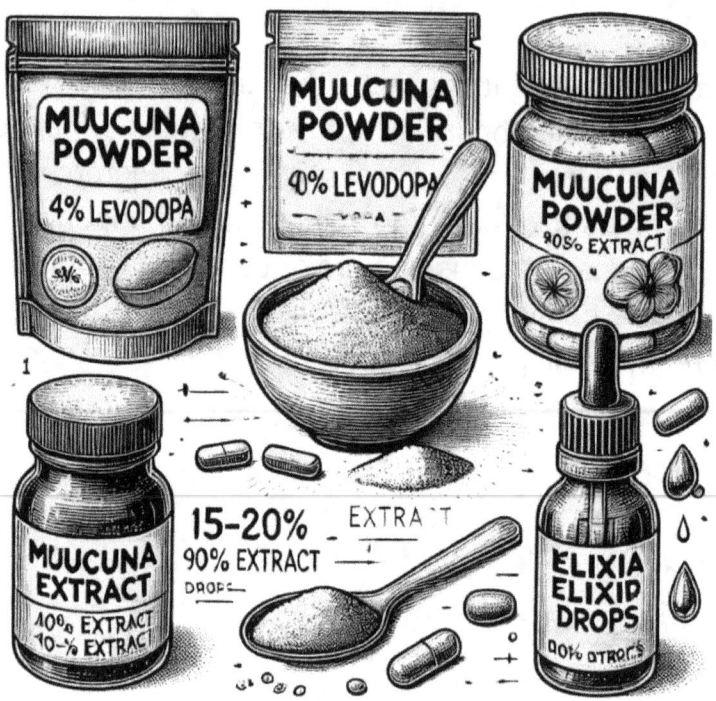

12. Mucuna preparation tables

Will follow the main brands grouped into the following sections:

PURE POWDER

PURE POWDER IN CAPSULES

EXTRACTS AT 15-25%

EXTRACTS AT 40-60%

ULTRA CONCENTRATED EXTRACTS

ELIXIRS

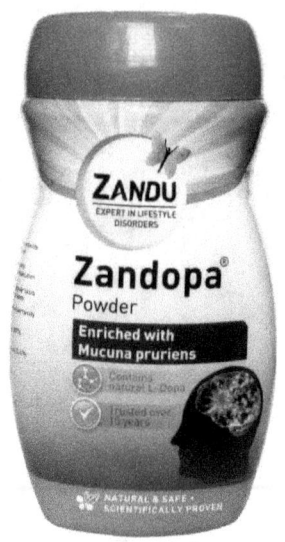
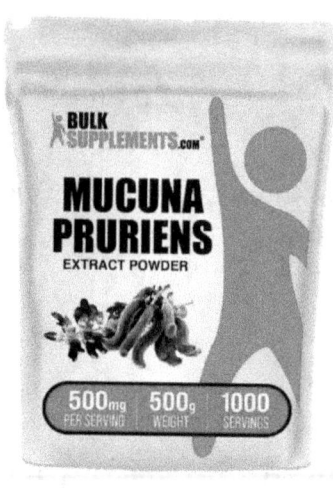
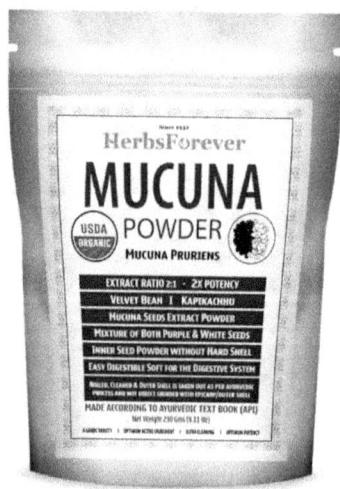
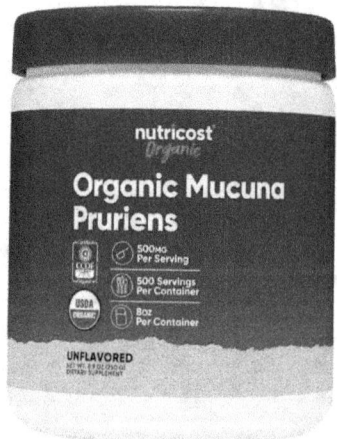

PURE POWDER

ZANDOPA	PURE POWDER	3.3 %	1 tsp = **100 mg** LD
	seeds	3 gr.	
BULK Supplements	PURE POWDER	4 %	1 tsp = **120 mg** LD
	seeds	3 gr.	
CARMEL Organics	PURE POWDER	4 %	1 tsp = **120 mg** LD
	seeds	3 gr.	
NOVA Nutritions	PURE POWDER	4 %	1 tsp = **120 mg** LD
	seeds	3 gr.	
NUTRICOST	PURE POWDER	4 %	1 tsp = **120 mg** LD
	seeds	3 gr.	
BANYAM	PURE POWDER	4.5 %	1 tsp = **135 mg** LD
	seeds	3 gr.	
HERBS Forever	PURE POWDER	4.75 %	1 tsp = **142 mg** LD
	seeds	3 gr.	

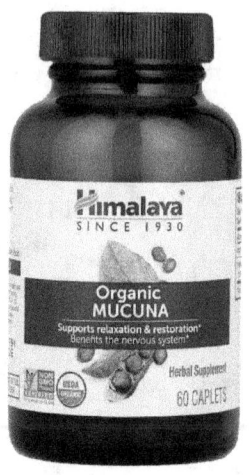
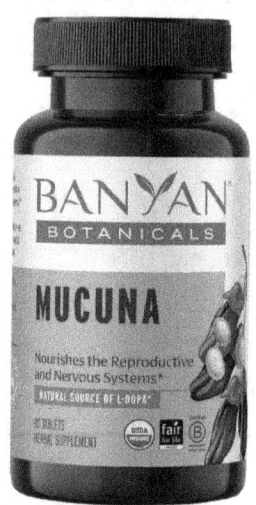
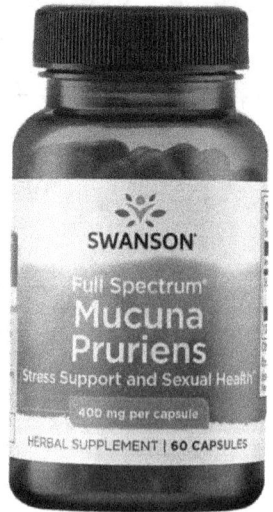
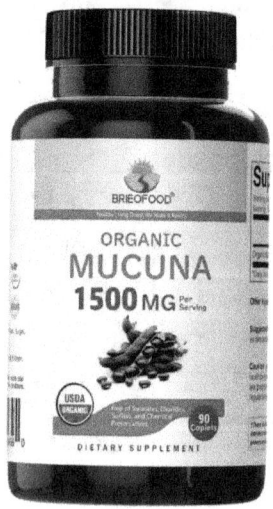

PURE POWDER IN CAPSULES OR TABLETS

HIMALAYA	Capsule PURE POWDER	0.25 and 4 %	1 caps = **11 mg** LD
	stem and seeds	600 mg	

SWANSON	Capsule PURE POWDER	4 %	1 caps = **16 mg** LD
	seeds	400 mg	

SUPREME	Capsule PURE POWDER	4 %	1 caps = **20 mg** LD
	seeds	490 mg	

BANYAN	Tablet PURE POWDER	4.5 %	1 caps = **22 mg** LD
	seeds	500 mg	

BRIEOFOOD	Tablet PURE POWDER	4 %	1 caps= **30 mg** LD
	seeds	750 mg	

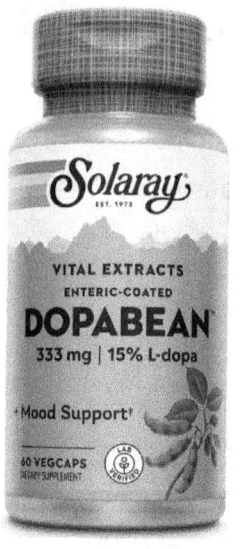
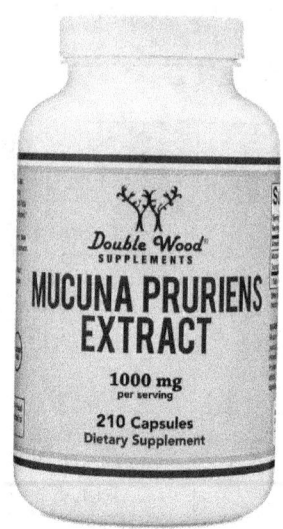
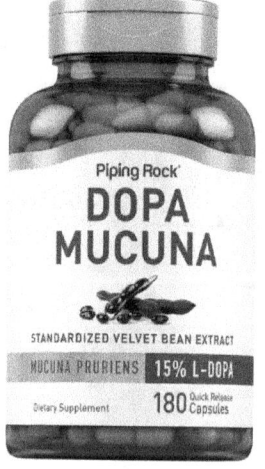
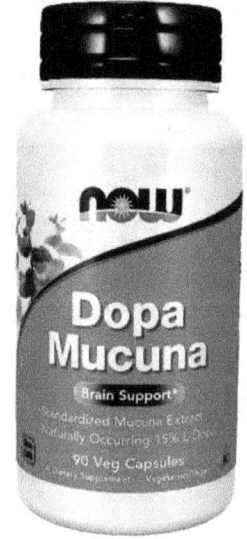

EXTRACT CAPSULES 15-25 %

PURE Encapsulations	Capsule EXTRACT	15 %	1 caps = **10 mg** LD
	seeds + B6 + tea	66 mg	
ADVANCE Physician	Capsule EXTRACT	15 %	1 caps = **30 mg** LD
	seeds	200 mg	
SOLARAY Dopabean	Capsule EXTRACT	15 %	1 caps = **50 mg** LD
	seeds	333 mg	
PIPING ROCK	Capsule EXTRACT	15 %	1 caps = **52 mg** LD
	seeds	350 mg	
NOW Dopamucuna	Capsule EXTRACT	15 %	1 caps = **60 mg** LD
	seeds	400 mg	
BONUSAN	Capsule EXTRACT	15 %	1 caps = **60 mg** LD
	seeds	400 mg	
DOUBLE WOODS	Capsule EXTRACT	20 %	1 caps = **100 mg** LD
	seeds	500 mg	
ZAZZEE	Capsule EXTRACT	20 %	1 caps = **100 mg** LD
	seeds	500 mg	

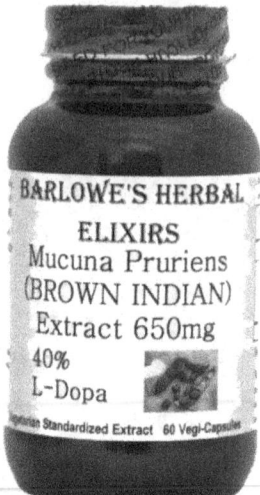
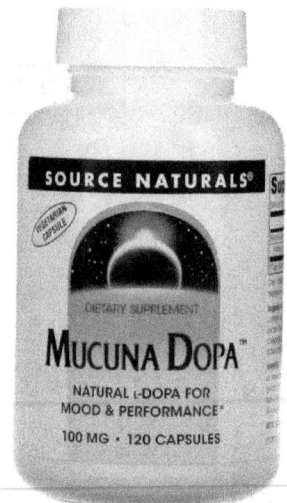
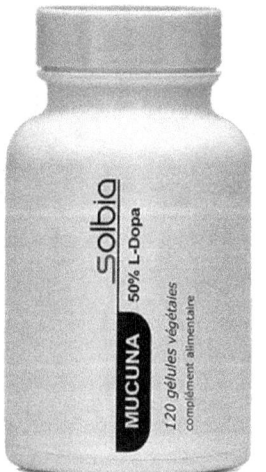
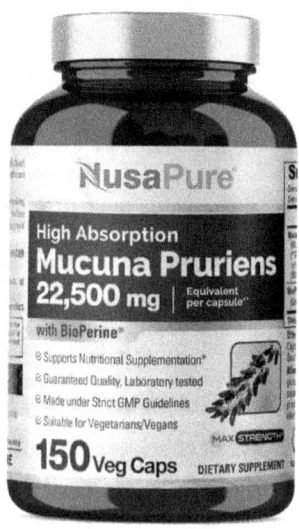

EXTRACT CAPSULES 40-60%

BIOVEA	Capsule EXTRACT	40 %	1 caps = **100 mg** LD
	seeds	*250 mg*	
NUTRICOST	Capsule EXTRACT	40 %	1 caps = **160 mg** LD
	seeds	*400 mg*	
HEALTH Essentials	Capsule EXTRACT	40% + 4%	1 caps = **190 mg** LD
	seeds	*700 mg*	
BARLOWE	Capsule EXTRACT	40 %	1 capsule = **260 mg** LD
	seeds	*650 mg*	
SOLBIA	Capsule EXTRACT	50 %	1 caps = **100 mg** LD
	Seeds	200 mg	
HERBAL Powers	Capsule EXTRACT	60 %	1 caps = **60 mg** LD
	seeds	*100 mg*	
SOURCE Naturals	Capsule EXTRACT	60 %	1 caps = **100 mg** LD
	seeds	*166 mg*	
NUSAPURE	Capsule EXTRACT	40 %	1 caps = **180 mg** LD
	seeds + piperine	*450 mg*	

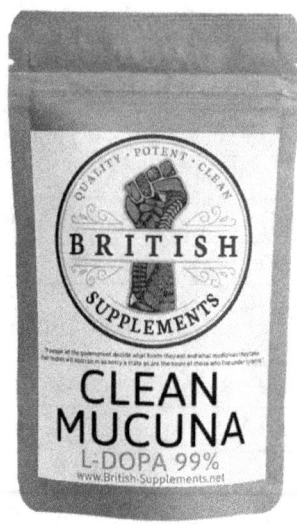
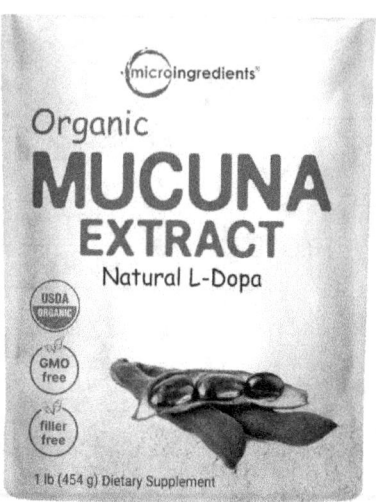
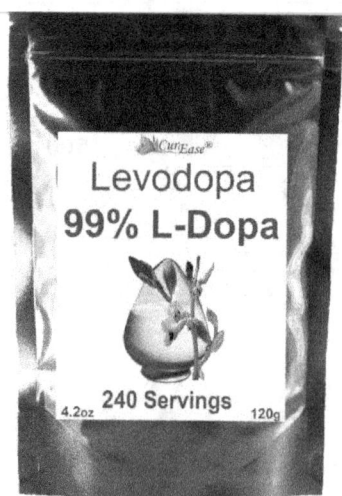
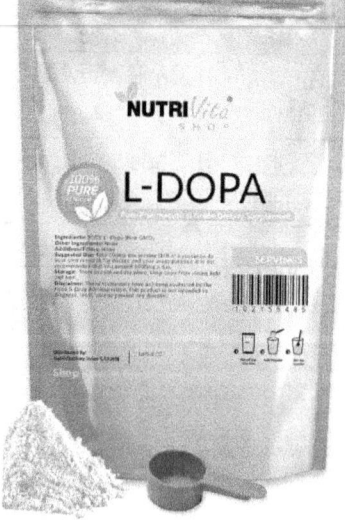

ULTRA-CONCENTRATED > 90 %

MICROINGREDIENTS	Powder EXTRACt 20:1	% ?	1 tsp = **120 mg** LD?
	seeds	cup 250 mg?	
BRITISH Supplements	Capsule EXTRACT	99 %	1 caps = **237 mg** LD
	seeds	240 mg	
BRITISH Suppl HIGH	Capsule EXTRACT	99 %	1 caps = **353 mg** LD
	seeds	357 mg	
BRITISH Supplements	Powder EXTRACT	99 %	1 tsp = **2970 mg** ?
	seeds	cup 1/8	
CUREASE	Powder EXTRACT	99 %	1 tsp = **2970 mg** ?
	seeds	cup 1/8	
NUTRIVITA	Powder EXTRACT	100 %	1 tsp = **2970 mg**?
	seeds	3 g	

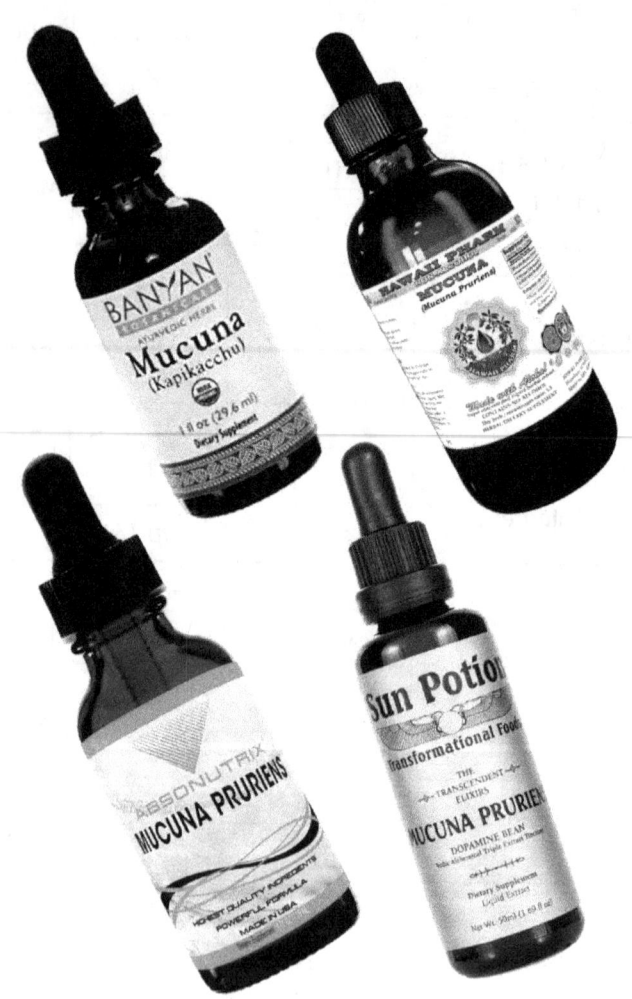

ELIXIRS AND TINCTURES

	Elixir EXTRACT 1:3	4 %	1 ml = **12 mg** LD
HAWAI Pharm	seeds	300 mg	

	Elixir EXTRACT 1:3-4	4 %	1 ml = **13 mg** LD
HERBAL TERRA	seeds	333 mg	

	Elixir EXTRACT 1:3	4.5 %	1 ml = **15 mg** LD
BANYAN	seeds	333 mg	

	Elixir EXTRACT 1:?	4 %	1 ml = **39 mg** LD?
ABSONUTRIX	seeds	982 mg?	

Bibliography

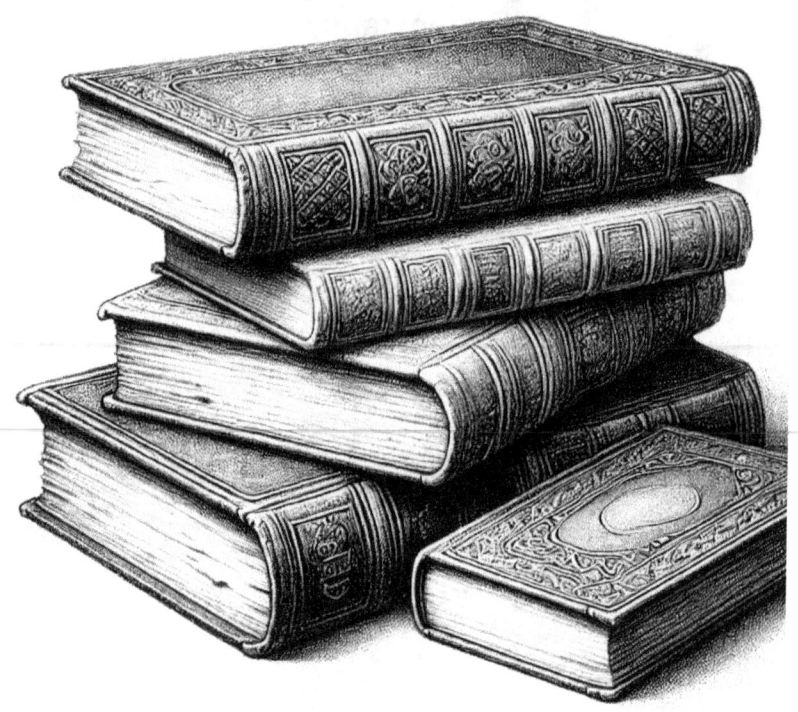

Boonmongkol TH et al. Systematic review of Mucuna Pruriens as a treatment for Parkinson's disease. Mov Disord 2019; 34 (suppl 2). https://www. mdsabstracts. org/abstract/systematic-re view-of-mucuna-pruriens-as-a-treatment-for-parkinsons-disease/.

Caronni S, Cilia R et al. Mucuna pruriens to treat Parkinson's disease in low-income countries: Recommendations and practical guidelines from the farmer to clinical trials. Paving the way for future use in clinical practice. Parkinsonism Relat Disord. 2024; 124:106983.

Cassani E, Cilia R, Laguna J et al. Mucuna pruriens for Parkinson's disease: Low-cost preparation method, laboratory measures and pharmacokinetics profile. J Neurol Sci. 2016; 365:175-180.

Cilia R, Laguna J, Pezzoli G. Daily intake of Mucuna pruriens in advanced Parkinson's disease: A 16-week, noninferiority, randomized, crossover, pilot study . Parkinsonism Relat Disord. 2018; 49: 60-66.

Cilia R, Laguna J, Cassani E et al. *Mucuna pruriens* in Parkinson's disease: A double-blind, randomized, controlled, crossover study . Neurology. 2017; 89:432-438.

Cohen PA, Ayula B, Katragunta K, Khan I. Levodopa Content of Mucuna pruriens Supplements in the NIH Dietary Supplement Label Database. JAMA Neurol. 2022; 79:1085-1086.

Contin M, Lopane G, Passini A, Poli F, Iannello C, Guarino. Mucuna pruriens in Parkinson Disease: A Kinetic-Dynamic Comparison with Levodopa Standard Formulations. Clin Neuropharmacol. 2015; 38.

Danique L M Radder, Andreas T Tiel Groenestege, Inge Boers[1], Eline W Muilwijk[2], Bastiaan R Bloem. Mucuna Pruriens Combined with Carbidopa in Parkinson's Disease: A Case Report. J Parkinsons Dis. 2019; 9:437-439.

González Maldonado R. Mucuna versus Parkinson's disease. Create Space (Amazon), North Charleston 2014.

González Maldonado R. Natural remedies for Parkinson's disease. Create Space (Amazon), North Charleston 2017.

González-Maldonado R, González-Redondo R, Di Caudo C. Benefits of the combination of Mucuna, green tea and levodopa/benserazide in Parkinson's disease. Rev Neurol. 2016; 62:525-526. (Article in Spanish)

González-Maldonado R, González-Redondo R, Di Caudo C. The clinical effects of mucuna and green tea in combination with levodopa-benserazide in advanced Parkinson's disease: Experience from a case report. International Parkinson and Movement Disorders Society, Berlin June 2016. Mov Disord 2016; 31 Suppl 2, pp. S639.

Hinz M, Stein A, Cole T. The Parkinson's disease death rate: carbidopa and vitamin B6. Clin Pharmacol. 2014. (a); 6: 161–169. doi:10.2147/CPAA.S70707

Hinz M, Stein A, Cole T. Parkinson's disease: carbidopa, nausea, and dyskinesia. Clin Pharmacol. 2014. (b); 6:189-94. doi: 10.2147/ CPAA.S72234.

Hu X, et al. Piperine improves levodopa availability in the 6-OHDA-lesioned rat model of Parkinson's disease by suppressing gut bacterial tyrosine decarboxylase. CNS Neurosci Ther. 2024; 30: e14383.

Katzenschlager R, Lees AJ. Treatment of Parkinson's di-sease: levodopa as the first choice. J Neurol. 2002; 249 Suppl 2: II19-24.

Katzenschlager R, Evans A, Manson A, Patsalos PN, Ratnaraj N, Watt H, Timmermann L, Van der Giessen R, Lees AJ. Mucuna pruriens in Parkinson's disease: a double blind clinical and pharmacological study. J Neurol Neurosurg Psychiatry. 2004; 75:1672-1677.

doi:10.1136/ jnnp 2003.028761.PMID : 15548480 Free PMC article. Clinical Trial.

Lieu CA, Venkiteswaran K, Gilmour TP, Rao AN, Petticoffer AC, Gilbert EV, Deogaonkar M, Manyam BV, Subramanian T. The Antiparkinsonian and Antidys-kinetic Mechanisms of Mucuna pruriens in the MPTP-Treated Nonhuman Primate. Evid Based Complement Alternat Med. 2012; 2012:840247.

Nagashima Y, Kondo T, Sakata M, Koh J, Ito H. Effects of soybean ingestion on pharmacokinetics of levodopa and motor symptoms of Parkinson's disease--In relation to the effects of Mucuna pruriens. J Neurol Sci. 2016; 361:229-34.

Manyam B. An Alternative Medicine Treatment for Parkinson's Disease: Results of a Multicenter Clinical Trial (HP-200). The Journal of Alternative and Complementary Medicine. 1995; 1:249-255.

Manyam BV, Sanchez-Ramos JR. Traditional and complementary therapies in Parkinson's disease. Adv Neurol.1999; 80:565-574.

Olanow CW, Torti M, Kieburtz K et al. Continuous versus intermittent oral administration of levodopa in Parkinson's disease patients with motor fluctuations: A pharmacokinetics, safety, and efficacy study. Mov Disord.2019; 34:425-429.

Pathak-Gandhi N, Vaidya AD. Management of Parkinson's disease in Ayurveda: Medicinal plants and adjuvant measures. J Ethnopharmacol. 2017 : 197 :46-51.

Soumyanath A, Denne T, Hiller A et al. Analysis of Levodopa Content in Commercial Mucuna pruriens Products Using High-Performance Liquid Chromatography with Fluorescence Detection. J Alt Compl Med 2018; 24:182-186.

Timmermann L, Van der Giessen R, Lees AJ. Mucuna pruriens in Parkinson's disease: a double blind clinical and pharmacological study. J Neurol Neurosurg Psychiatry. 2004 Dec;75(12):1672-7.

Van der Giessen R, Olanow W, Lees A, Wagner H. Pharmaceutical compositions and uses comprising Mucuna Pruriens seed powder and extracts thereof in the treatment of neurological diseases. International Application published under the Patent Cooperation Treaty, 2004 May 13. WO 2004/039385 A2, PCT/EP2003/010975. https: //register.epo.org/ ipfw retrieve?apn = JP. 2004547503. A&lng =en

Table of contents

Introduction..9

1. Mucuna is more than just levodopa 13

    UNKNOWN COMPONENTS IN MUCUNA 14

    IMPROVEMENTS IN MICE 14

        Essay 1. A traditional, very effective preparation 15

        Study 2: Rapid and lasting improvement 16

        Study 3: Comparison of high and low doses 17

        Study 4: High doses in advanced patients. 17

    OTHER ADVANTAGES OF MUCUNA 18

    QUADRUPLE THE DOSE..18

    MUCUNA WITH CARBIDOPA.................................19

    THE VOLUME PROBLEM 20

    PATENTS ON MUCUNA EXTRACTS 20

    DYSKINESIAS DUE TO LEVODOPA OR CARBIDOPA? 21

    CONTRAINDICATIONS AND WARNINGS 21

    PATIENTS DO NOT KNOW WHAT THEY ARE TAKING 22

SKEPTICAL DOCTORS 22

CONCLUSIONS 23

2. The "mucuna of the poor" 25

CULTIVATION IN UNDERDEVELOPED COUNTRIES 25

MEDICINAL USE.. 26

PREPARATION TO ELIMINATE TOXINS 26

HEALTH EFFECTS AND SAFETY OF USE 26

MUCUNA FOR POOR PATIENTS........................... 27

CONCLUSIONS 28

3. The "Internet mucuna"................................ 31

SUSTAINABLE CROPS AND HARVESTING 31

TRADITIONAL AND MODERN PROCESSING 31

QUALITY CONTROL AND STANDARDIZATION 32

LEVODOPA VARIES ACCORDING TO PROCESSING 33

PACKAGING AND PRESERVATION....................... 33

BIOTECHNOLOGY 33

ETHICS AND FAIR TRADE 34

CONCENTRATED SEED EXTRACTS 34

EXTRACTION TECHNIQUES................................. 34

NORMALIZATION (STANDARDIZATION) 35

ENCAPSULATION AND FORMULATION................ 35

QUALITY CONTROL	35
INTERNET SCAMS WITH MUCUNA	36
TIPS WHEN BUYING MUCUNA	37

4. Pure seeds or whole plant powder 41

PURE MUCUNA SEEDS POWDER	41
PURE POWDER CAPSULES	42
MUCUNA STEMS AND LEAVES POWDER	42
LEVODOPA PERCENTAGE	43
CONCENTRATIONS RANGE	43
BIOAVAILABILITY, DOSAGE	44
DO NOT DOSE WITH SPOONS	45
PURE SEED POWDER BRANDS	46
ZANDOPA powder - *zanducare.com*	48
BULKSUPPLEMENTS powder - *bulksupplements.com*	49
CARMEL Organics powder - *bulksupplements.com*	50
NOVA NUTRITIONS powder - *bulksupplements.com*	51
NUTRICOST powder - *nutricost.com*	52
KAPIKACCHU powder - *banyanbotanicals.com*	53
HERBS FOREVER powder . *herbsforever.com*	54
PURE POWDER IN CAPSULES OR TABLETS	55
HIMALAYA organic - *iherbs.com*	56
SWANSON capsules powder – *swansoneurope.com*	57

SUPREME capsules powder – *supremenaturals.com* **58**

BANYAN tablets - *banyanbotanicals.com* **59**

BRIEOFOOD capsules powder – *brieofood.com* **60**

5.   **Low-concentrated extracts**¡Error! Marcador no definido.

   THE PROCEDURE 63

      1. Selection and Drying 63

      2. Fine Grinding 64

      3. Extraction of Bioactive Components 64

      4. Filtration and Concentration 65

      5. Standardization (Normalization) 65

      6. Encapsulation or Formulation 65

      7. Quality Control 66

   TYPES OF EXTRACTS 66

      Mucuna Liquid Extracts 66

      Mucuna Extracts Powder 67

      Standard and Complex Extracts 67

      Ultra-concentrated extracts 68

      Extracts in Capsules: Convenience and Precision .. 68

   CHOOSING THE RIGHT PRODUCT 69

   CHOOSING THE RIGHT DOCTOR 69

   RANGE OF THERAPEUTIC APPLICATIONS 70

   MOST POPULAR BRANDS 70

ETTA VITA - *ettavita.com* 72
PURE ENCAPSULATIONS - *pureencapsulations.com* ... 73
ADVANCE PHYSICIAN - *physicianformulas.com* 74
SOLARAY Dopabean – *solaray.com* 75
HORBÄACH - *pipingrock.com* 76
PIPING ROCK - *pipingrock.com* 77
DOPA MUCUNA NOW - *nowfoods.com* 78
BONUSAN mucuna – *bonusan.com* 79
DOUBLE WOOD - *doublewood.com* 80
ZAZZEE - *zazzeenaturals.com* 81
KETER Wellness - *keterwellness.com* 82
VITAKRUID – *vitakruid.nl* 83
MACUDOPA - *macudopausa.com* 84
HERBSFOREVER - *herbsforever.com* 85

6. **Medium-concentrated extracts (40-60%)** ... 87

HEALTH Essent.-*healthessentialsdirect.co.uk.com* 91
BARLOWE -*barloweherbalelixirs.com*.........................92
SOLBIA – *en.solbia.com* 93
HERBAL POWERS MP – *herbal powers.com* 94
SOURCE NATURALS MDopa - *sourcenaturals.com* 95
NUSAPURE - *nusapure.com*.. 96

7. **Ultra-concentrated extracts (>90%)** 99

RISK OF OVERDOSE 99

USEFUL IN ADVANCED CASES 100

CHEMICAL EXTRACTION METHODS 100

WHAT IS LEFT OF THE PLANT? 100

OVERDOSE EUPHORIA 101

MICROINGREDIENTS – microingredients.com 102

BRITISH SUPPLEMENTS - britishsupplements . *net* 104

BRITISH SUPPLEMENTS - britishsupplements . *net* 105

CUREASE - *curease.com* 106

NUTRIVITA POWDER NUTRIVITA.SHOP.COM 107

8. Liquid extracts (elixirs) 109

ELIXIR OF SEEDS OR THE WHOLE PLANT 109

PROCESS FOR MUCUNA ELIXIR 110

ELIXIR AND TINCTURE: DIFFERENCES 113

COMMERCIAL ELIXIRS AND TINCTURES OF MUCUNA 113

HAWAI PHARM Elixir - *hawaiipharm.com* 114

BANYAN Elixir – *banyanbotanicals.com* 116

9. How to start with mucuna ! 121

MUCUNA INDIVIDUAL PROFILE 121

WHAT INFLUENCES THE METABOLISM OF MUCUNA 121

VARIABLE RESPONSE ACCORDING TO MUCUNA 123

VARIOUS PRESENTATIONS OF MUCUNA 123

THE OTHER COMPONENTS 124

CHOOSING THE MOST APPROPRIATE MUCUNA 124

PRACTICAL CASES 124

PURE SEED POWDER (NO EXTRACTS) 125

SEED POWDER CAPSULES 127

POWDER AND EXTRACTS IN CAPSULES 128

MONITOR THE RESPONSE 130

DOSE ADJUSTMENTS IN PERIODIC CONSULTATIONS 131

MONOTHERAPY WITH MUCUNA 131

INCREASED DOSE OF MUCUNA 133

CONTROL RESPONSE AND TOLERANCE 134

ADD GREEN TEA TO MUCUNA 134

MUCUNA WITH CARBIDOPA ALONE¡Error! Marcador no definido.

MUCUNA WITH A LITTLE SINEMET 137

QUARTER OF MADOPAR OR HALF SINEMET PLUS? .. 138

10. **Combining mucuna and drugs 141**

PREVIOUS STEPS 142

CONSIDER THE INDIVIDUAL RESPONSE 142

SMALL DOSES AND PERIODIC ADJUSTMENTS 143

DOPAMINERGIC AGONISTS 143

CONTINUOUS MONITORING 143

PART OF LEVODOPA MAY BE FLEXIBLE 144

PRACTICAL CASES... 144
11. Patients lose their patience (Patient Forum) . 157
WIDESPREAD DISCONTENT...................................... 157
MUCUNA: SALVATION OR FALSE HOPE?...............158
WHY HIDE WHAT WORKS?....................................... 159
AN UNDERVALUED SOURCE OF KNOWLEDGE 160
CALL TO ACTION 160
CONCLUSIONS 161
12. Mucuna preparation tables 163
Bibliography 177

Finis

www.ingramcontent.com/pod-product-compliance
Lightning Source LLC
Chambersburg PA
CBHW052154220526
45471CB00004B/1669